THE SCIENCE OF WELL-BEING

Wallace D. Wattles
and
Dr. Judith Powell

TOP OF THE MOUNTAIN PUBLISHING
Largo, Florida 34643-5117 U.S.A.

For a FREE Catalog, write, phone or fax:
Top Of The Mountain Publishing
11

I
FREE Catalog, Write, Phone or Fax
TOP OF THE MOUNTAIN PUBLISHING
BOX 2244 PINELLAS PARK, FL 33780-2244
Fax 813 391-4598 - Tel 813 391-3958
Web Site http://www.abcinfo.com

Copyright 1993 by Dr. Judith Powell

Library of Congress Cataloging Publication Data
Wattles, Wallace Delois, 1860 - 1911
The science of well-being/ by Wallace D. Wattles & Ju-
dith Powell.
p. cm.
Rev. ed. of: The science of being well. 1910.
ISBN 1-56087-059-1 (pbk.): $8.95
1. New Thought. 2. Mental healing. 3. Health. I.
Powell, Judith L., 1957 -   . II. Wattles, Wallace
Delois, 1860-1911. Science of being well. III Title.
BF639.W352 1993 158'.1—dc20   93-17454CIP

Manufactured in the United States of America

CONTENTS

FOREWORD

It is so strange that we learn so many unnecessary tidbits in school, and almost totally neglect to educate ourselves on the practical basics about the human body-machine which must see us through all of our days. Much of the world's misery is due to ignorance of the ABC's of Health. The world's society perpetuates fear, worry and anxiety... these stressful emotions consume our energies, and are therefore, the true enemies of relaxation, happiness, and peace of mind. All of these mental pressures result from our lack of knowledge on how to naturally maintain our health.

Health is not a condition of matter, but of mind. Good health depends primarily upon right thinking and congruent right habits of living. If you want to live long and be healthy and active, you should continually keep your body and brain active by doing all your duties, while striving for excellence. By learning and applying the Principles of Health in your eating, drinking, breathing, and sleeping habits, you can live a long and youthful existence.

The Science of Well-Being will guide you to cultivate an awareness of those activities which you do every day. Take note of how you sit, walk, eat, breathe, and any other habitual action. Remember, the important thing is not what you do occasionally, but what you do daily. The Buddhists say if you neglect to be aware of your physical actions, it makes spiritual exercises ineffective. Become conscious of your bodily actions as well as your thought processes.

Our body is made up of what we breathe, drink, and eat (in that order of importance). When we furnish it with the necessary requirements for growth and repair, the human body is designed to produce all the needed energy over an amazingly long period of time. If you take even reasonable care of your body, using the common-sense basics in this book, your body will produce an amazing energy flow and sustain itself in general good health. *However, to treat the body without giving attention to the mind, is effort wasted and energy exhausted.*

Balanced living — which is thought and action working together for a total Conception of Health — is the true key to maintaining health, strength, and beauty.

Enjoy your newly-found energy... your health... and a full life!

Judith Powell

PREFACE

*T*his volume is the third of a series, the first of which is *The Science of Getting Rich,* the second in the trilogy of which is *The Science of Becoming Excellent.* As the first book is intended solely for those who want money, and the second is for those who desire to reach the top of their potential toward excellence, so this book in your hands is for those who want health, and who want a practical guide and handbook, not a philosophical treatise. It is an instructor in the use of the *Universal Principle of Life.* Our efforts are to explain the principles in such a plain and simple fashion that you (though you may have given no previous study to New Thought, metaphysics, or medicine), may readily follow it to perfect health.

While retaining all the fundamental elements, we have carefully eliminated all non-essentials; we have used no technical, obtuse, or difficult language, and have kept the one point in view at all times. As its title asserts, the book deals with science, not speculation. The *Monastic Theory of the Universe* — the theory that matter, mind, consciousness, and life are all manifestations of *one* Substance — is now accepted by most philosophical thinkers. If you accept this theory, you cannot deny the logical conclusions you will find here. Good health depends primarily upon the right way of thinking (Part I of this book), followed by the right habits of eating, drinking, breathing, and sleeping (Parts II & III of this book).

We can say of *The Science of Well-Being* that it works; and wherever its laws are complied with, it can no more fail to work than the science of geometry can fail to work. *If the tissues of your body have not been so destroyed that continued life is impossible, you can get well;* and if you will think and act in a Certain Way, you will get well. If you wish to fully understand the *Monastic Theory of the Cosmos*, you are recommended to read Hegel and Emerson.

Don't make the mistake of studying many conflicting theories, and practicing, at the same time, parts of several different "systems"; for if you get well, it must be by giving your WHOLE MIND to the right way of thinking and living. Remember, *The Science of Well-Being* provides a complete and sufficient guide in every aspect of health. Concentrate upon the way of thinking and acting this book prescribes, follow it in every detail, and you will get well; or if you are already well, you will remain so.

Trusting that you will go on until the price-less blessing of perfect health as yours, I remain...

Very Truly Yours
W D Wattles

MEDICAL DISCLAIMER

The intention of this book is to provide a simple program of health — with suggestions on how to eat, sleep, breathe, and exercise.

Its message is for complete mental and physical health — an inspirational guide to well-being. It is our efforts to provide a spiritual and mental path towards overall health.

Under no circumstances should this book and its contents and/or message be used as a complete medical reference. If you suspect and/or are in need of medical treatment, we urge you to consult your physician.

The methods, techniques, and practices regarding diet, eating, exercise, sleeping, and breathing suggested in this book are best associated in conjunction with the advice of a physician.

If, at any time, you feel discomfort, pain or abnormal health as a result of these suggestions, cease activity and consult a physician immediately.

PART I

THE HEALING POWER OF BELIEF AND WILL

THE 12 WARNING SIGNS OF HEALTH

1. Persistent presence of support network.
2. Chronic positive expectations; tendency to frame events in a constructive light.
3. Episodic peak experiences.
4. Sense of spiritual involvement.
5. Increased sensitivity.
6. Tendency to adapt to changing conditions.
7. Rapid response and recovery of adrenaline system due to repeated challenges.
8. Increased appetite for physical activity.
9. Tendency to identify and communicate feelings.
10. Repeated episodes of gratitude, generosity or related emotions.
11. Compulsion to contribute to society.
12. Persistent sense of humor.

If five or more of these indicators are present, you may be at risk for full-blown health!

Brain/Mind Bulletin
Los Angeles, CA
March 1993 Issue

CHAPTER ONE

THE PRINCIPLE OF HEALTH

*W*e have only one body in which to live out our days to the fullest. And nothing will aid us so well in attaining success and excellence in life, as will keeping ourselves in perfect physical condition. Nothing in life can mean more to us than our health... staying in top physical form for the fullest expression of the Source within us.

To Quote Mahatma Gandhi, "One of the greatest investments which we can make is to invest in health, for there is no other investment like it. It increases our efficiency, our effectiveness in life, our creative and productive ability. Health is life insurance... success and happiness insurance."

To begin our healthful journey, certain fundamental truths must be known in the beginning, and accepted without question, in the personal application of *The Science of Well-Being*, as in the first two books of this series. Some of these truths we state here:

The perfectly natural performance of function constitutes health; and the perfectly natural performance of function results from the natural action of the *Principle of Life*.

> ✳ *TRUTH*: There is a *Principle of Life* in the Universe; it is the one Living Substance from which all things are made. This Living Substance permeates, penetrates, and fills the interspaces of the Universe; it is in and through all things, like a very refined and diffusible ether. All life comes from *It*; *Its* life is all the life

there is. Humans are one form of this Living Substance, and we have within us a *Principle of Health. (The word Principle is used to mean Source.)*

✳ *TRUTH:* The *Principle of Health* in you, when in full constructive activity, causes all the voluntary functions of your life to be perfectly performed. It is the *Principle of Health* within you which really works all healing, no matter what "system" or "remedy" is employed. *This Principle of Health is brought into Constructive Activity by thinking in a Certain Way.*

We proceed now to prove this last statement. We all know cures are brought about by all the different, and often *opposite,* methods employed in the various branches of the healing art.

The allopath, who gives a strong dose of a counter-poison, cures his patient; and the homeopath, who gives a wee dose of the poison most similar to that of the disease, also cures it.

If allopathy ever cured any given disease, it is certain that homeopathy never cured that disease;

> *... medicines, manipulations, prayers, foods and herbs, affirmations, and hygienic practices cure whenever they cause the Principle of Health to become active; and fail whenever they do not cause it to become active.*

and if homeopathy ever cured an ailment, allopathy could not possibly cure that ailment. The two systems are radically opposite in theory and practice, and yet both "cure" most diseases.

Even the remedies used by physicians in any one school are not the same. Go with a case of indigestion to half a dozen doctors, and compare their prescriptions; it is more than likely you will be prescribed many different medications. Must we not conclude that their patients are healed by a *Principle of Health* within themselves, and not by something in the varying "remedies"? Not only this, but we find the same ailments cured...

* by the osteopath with manipulations of the spine;
* by the faith healer with prayer;
* by the herbalist with food combinations and herbal remedies;
* by the Christian Scientist with a formulated creed statement;

16

✳ by the metaphysician with affirmation;
✳ by the hygienist with differing plans of living.

What conclusion can we come to in the face of all these facts? There is a *Principle of Health*, which is the same in all people, and which really accomplishes all the cures. There is something in all the "systems" which, *under favorable conditions, arouses the Principle of Health to ACTION.* That is, medicines, manipulations, prayers, foods and herbs, affirmations, and hygienic practices *cure whenever they cause the Principle of Health to become active;* and fail whenever they do not cause it to become active. Does not all this indicate that the *results depend upon the way the patient thinks about the remedy, rather than upon the ingredients in the prescription?*

There is an old story which quite powerfully illustrates this point. It is said that in the Middle Ages, the bones of a saint, kept in one of the monasteries, were working miracles of healing. On certain days, a great crowd of the afflicted gathered to touch the relics, and all who did so were healed. On the eve of one of these occasions, some sacrilegious rascal gained access to the case

> *The Power which heals is in the patient themselves. Whether it will become active or not does not depend upon the physical or mental means used, but upon the way the patient THINKS about these means.*

in which the wonder-working relics were kept, and stole the bones. In the morning, with the usual crowd of sufferers waiting at the gates, the fathers found themselves without the source of the miracle-working power. They resolved to keep the matter quiet, hoping by doing so, they might find the thief and recover their treasure.

Hastening to the cellar of the convent, they dug up the bones of a murderer, who had been buried there many years before. These they placed in the case, intending to make some plausible excuse for the failure of the saint to perform his usual miracles on this particular day; and then they let in the waiting assemblage of the sick and afflicted. To the intense astonishment of those in on the secret, the bones of the criminal proved as effective as those of the saint!... and the healing went on as before. One of the fathers is said to have left a history of the occurrence, in which he confessed that, in his judgment, the healing power had been in the people themselves all the time, and never in the bones at all.

Whether the story is true or not, the conclusion applies to all the cures brought by all the healing systems. *The Power which heals is in the patient themselves. Whether it will become active or not does not depend upon the physical or mental means used, but upon the way the patient THINKS about these means.* There is a *Universal Principle of Life,* as Jesus taught; a great spiritual Healing Power; and there is a *Principle of Health* in you which is related to this Healing Power. This is dormant or active, according to the way you think. *You can always quicken it into activity by thinking in a Certain Way.*

✳ Your getting well does not depend upon the *adoption of some system,* or the finding of some system, or the finding of some remedy — people with your identical ailments have been healed by all systems and all remedies.

✳ It does not depend upon *climate;* some people are well and others are sick in all climates.

---

* It does not depend upon *vocation*, unless in the case of those who work under poisonous conditions; people are well in all trades and professions.

* *Your getting well depends upon your beginning to THINK and ACT in a Certain Way.* The way you think about things is determined by what you believe about them.

Your thoughts are determined by your faith, and the results depend upon your making a personal application of your faith. If you have faith in the effectiveness of a medicine, and are able to apply this faith to yourself, the medicine will certainly cause you to be cured... but though your faith be great, you will not be cured unless you *apply it to yourself.* Many sick people have faith for others, but none in themselves! So, if you have faith in a system of diet, and can personally apply that faith, it will cure you; and if you have faith in prayers and affirmations, and personally apply your faith, prayers and affirmations will cure you.

SUMMARY

Faith, personally applied, cures. However, no matter how great the belief or how persistent the thought, it will not cure without personal application. *The Science of Well-Being,* then, includes the two fields of THOUGHT and ACTION. In order to be well, it is not enough to merely think in a Certain Way — *you must apply your healing thoughts to yourself, and you must express and externalize it in your outward life by acting in the same way you think.*

To expect vigorous health and the enjoyment which it brings, and at the same time, live in open defiance of the Laws of Health, is to expect that which cannot take place. *You must be congruent in thought and action!*

CHAPTER TWO

THE FOUNDATIONS OF TRUE FAITH

*B*efore you can think in the Certain Way which will cause your disease or affliction to be healed, you must believe in certain truths:

> ✳ *TRUTH:* All things are made from one Living Substance, which, in its original state, permeates, penetrates, and fills the interspaces of the Universe.

While all visible things are made from It, this Substance, in Its first formless condition is in and through all the visible forms that It has made. Its life is in All, and Its intelligence is in All.

> ✳ *TRUTH*: Original Substance creates by thought, and Its method is by taking the form of that which It thinks about.

The thought of a form held by this Substance causes It to assume that form; the thought of a motion causes It to institute that motion. Forms are created by this Substance in moving Itself into certain attitudes or positions. When Original Substance wishes to create a given form, It thinks of the motions which will produce that form. When It wishes to create a world, It thinks of the motions, perhaps extending through ages, which will result in Its coming into the attitude and form of the world; and these motions are made.

For example, when It wishes to create an oak tree, It thinks of the sequence of movements, extending through time, which will result in the form of an oak tree; and these motions are made. The particular sequence of motions by which differing forms should be produced were established in the beginning; they are changeless. *Cer-*

tain motions instituted in the Formless Substance will forever produce certain formations.

> ✳ TRUTH: Your body is formed from the Original Substance, and is the result of certain motions, which first existed as thoughts of Original Substance.

The motions which produce, renew, and repair your body are called *functions*, and these functions are of two classes: voluntary and involuntary.

> ✳ *1. The INVOLUNTARY functions are under the control of the Principle of Health in humans,* and are performed in a perfectly healthy manner so long as the individual thinks in a Certain Way.
>
> ✳ *2. The VOLUNTARY functions of life are eating, drinking, breathing, and sleeping. These, entirely or in part, are under the direction of YOUR conscious mind;* and you can perform them in a perfectly healthy way if you will it. If you do not perform them in a healthy way, you cannot be well for very long.

> *The Original Substance holds only the thoughts of PERFECT motion; PERFECT and healthy function; complete life.*

So you can see, if you think in a Certain Way, and eat, drink, breathe, and sleep in a corresponding way... you will be well.

The involuntary functions of your life are under the direct control of the *Principle of Health*, and so long as you *think* in a perfectly healthy way, these functions are perfectly performed; for the action of the *Principle of Health* is largely directed by your conscious mind; by your thoughts.

You are a thinking center capable of originating thought; and as you do not know everything, you make mistakes and have misconceptions. Not knowing everything, you believe things to be true which are not true. You may hold in your thoughts the idea of diseased and abnormal functioning and *conditions*. In doing so, *you* distort the action of the *Principle of Health*, causing diseased and abnormal functioning and conditions within your own body. *The Original Substance holds only the thoughts of PERFECT motion; PERFECT and healthy function; complete life.*

The Great Infinite never thinks disease or imperfection. But for countless ages, human beings have held the thoughts of disease, abnormality, old

> ...advancement is the inevitable result of the very act of living. Increase is always the result of active living; whatever lives must live more and more.

age, and death. The perverted functioning which results from these thoughts has become a part of the misguided inheritance of the human race. Our ancestors have, for many generations, held imperfect ideas concerning human form and functioning; and *we begin life with a race-consciousness filled with impressions of imperfection and disease.* This is not natural, or a part of the plan of Nature. The intention of Nature is to begin with a healthy body, pure thoughts, and unbiased beliefs. Only then can we mentally and physically function in a complete and effective manner.

> ✳ *TRUTH: The purpose of Nature can be nothing else than the perfection of life. This we see from the very nature of life itself.*

It is the nature of life to continually advance toward more perfect living — *advancement is the inevitable result of the very act of living. Increase is always the result of active living; whatever lives must live more and more.* The seed, lying in the granary, has life, but it is not living. Put it into the soil and it becomes active by beginning to gather from the surrounding substance, and to build a plant form. The growing plant will eventually produce an increase; a seed family containing thirty, sixty, or a hundred seeds, each having as much life as the first.

> ✳ *TRUTH*: Life, by living, increases. Life cannot live without increasing, and the fundamental impulse of life is to live.

It is in response to this fundamental impulse that Original Substance works, and creates. God must live; and He cannot truly live except through you as you create and increase. In multiplying forms, He is moving on to continual life.

> ✳ *TRUTH*: The Universe is a Great Advancing Life. The purpose of Nature is the advancement of life toward perfection; toward perfect functioning. The purpose of Nature is perfect health.

The purpose of Nature, so far as you are concerned, is that you should continuously advance into more life, and progress toward perfect

> *The natural state of humans is a state of perfect health; and everything in us, and in Nature, tends toward health.*

life. You should live the most complete life possible in your present sphere of action. This path must be so, because That which lives in you is seeking more life.

Give a little child a pencil and paper, and they begin to draw crude figures — That which lives in them is trying to express Itself in art. Give a child a set of blocks, and they will try to build something — That which lives in them is seeking expression in architecture. Seat them at a piano, and they will try to draw harmony from the keys — That which lives in them is trying to express Itself in music. That which lives in you is always seeking to live more through your desires, innovations, creativity, and talents; and since It lives most when you are well, the *Principle of Nature* in you can seek only health. *The natural state of humans is a state of perfect health; and everything in us, and in Nature, tends toward health.*

Sickness can have no place in the thought of Original Substance. By Its own nature, Original Substance continually impels Itself toward the fullest and most perfect life; therefore, toward health. Humans, as we exist in the thoughts of the Formless Substance, have perfect health. Disease is abnormal or perverted function; motion imperfectly made, or made in the direction of imperfect life. Disease has no place in the thought of the Thinking Stuff.

> ✳ *TRUTH*: The Supreme Mind never thinks of disease. Disease was not created or ordained by God, or sent forth from Him. It is wholly a product of separate consciousness; of the individual thought of humans.

God, the Formless Substance, does not see disease, think disease, know disease, or recognize disease. Disease is recognized only by the thoughts of humans. *The Source thinks nothing but health.*

SUMMARY

From all the foregoing, we see that health is a fact or TRUTH in the Original Substance from which we are all formed; and disease is truly the functioning of imperfection. It results from the distorted thoughts of men and women, past and present. If human thoughts had always been those of perfect health, it would be impossible for us to be anything else but perfectly healthy now!

You, in perfect health, is the thought of Original Substance. You, in imperfect health, is the result of your own failure to think perfect health, and to perform the voluntary functions of life in a healthy way. Your thoughts effect your actions, which affect your health. *Recognize that you must control thought and action, and you are on your way to well-being. Learn how to master them and you have achieved complete wellness.*

Your first step must be to learn how to think perfect health; and your second step is to learn how to eat, drink, breathe, and sleep in a perfectly healthy way. If you take these two steps, you will certainly become well, and remain so.

CHAPTER THREE

QUICKEN THE LIFE PRINCIPLE

*T*he human body is the dwelling place of an Energy which renews it when worn; which eliminates waste or poisonous matter; and which repairs the body when broken or injured. This Energy we call *Life* or *Prana*. Life is not generated or produced within the body; *it* produces the body!

The seed which has been kept in the storehouse for years will grow when planted in the soil; it will produce a plant. But the life in the plant is not generated by its growing — in reverse, it is the life which makes the plant grow!

✳ *TRUTH:* The performance of function does not cause life; it is life which causes function to be performed. Life is first; function afterward.

✳ *TRUTH:* It is life which distinguishes organic from inorganic matter, but life is not produced after the organization of matter.

✳ *TRUTH:* Life is the principle or force which causes organization; it builds organisms.

✳ *TRUTH:* Life is a principle or force inherent in Original Substance; all life is One.

This Life Principle of the All is the *Principle of Health* within us, and becomes constructively active whenever we think in a Certain Way. Whoever, therefore, thinks in this Certain Way, will surely have perfect health, if their external functioning is in conformity with their inner-thought. The action must conform to the thought

— *they must be congruent.* You cannot hope to be well by thinking health, when you eat, drink, breathe, and sleep like a sick person.

The Universal Life Principle, then, is the *Principle of Health* in humans. It is one with Original Substance. There is one Original Substance from which all things are made; this Substance is alive, and Its life is the Principle of Life of the Universe. This Substance has created from Itself all the forms of organic life by thinking them, or by thinking the motions and functions which produce them.

Original Substance thinks only health, because It knows all truth; there is no truth which is not known in the Formless, which is All, and in all. It not only knows all truth, but It has all power; Its vital power is the source of all existing energy. A conscious life which knows all truths and which has all power cannot go wrong or function imperfectly. Knowing all, It knows too much to go wrong, and so the Formless cannot be diseased or think disease.

You are a form of this Original Substance, and have a separate consciousness of your own... but your consciousness is limited, and therefore, imperfect. By reason of your limited knowledge, you can and do think incorrectly, and so you cause

> *The diseased or imperfect functioning may not instantly result from an imperfect thought, but it is bound to come if the thought becomes habitual.*

perverted and imperfect functioning of your own body. Your knowledge is limited, therefore, you can go wrong. *The diseased or imperfect functioning may not instantly result from an imperfect thought, but it is bound to come if the thought becomes habitual.* Any thought continuously held by you cultivates the establishment of the corresponding condition in your body.

By lack of knowledge, you also fail to perform the voluntary functions of your life in a healthy way. You do not know why, what, and how to eat; you know little about breathing, and less about sleep. You do all these things in a wrong way, and under wrong conditions; and illness results because you have neglected to follow the only sure guide to the knowledge of life. You have tried to live by logic rather than by instinct; you have made living a matter of art, and not of nature. Therefore, you have gone wrong.

Your only remedy is to begin to go right; and this cure you can surely do by thought, recognition, acceptance and action! It is the work of this book to teach the whole truth, so the individual who reads it will know too much to go wrong!

Your only remedy is to begin to go right; and this cure you can surely do by thought, recognition, acceptance and action!

The thoughts of disease produce the forms of disease. You must learn to think health. Taking on the thought and form of Original Substance, you will then become the reflection of health, and manifest the perfection of well-being in all your functioning.

All the sick who have been healed, by whatsoever "system," have thought in a Certain Way. A little examination will show us what this Way truly is.

✳ The people who were healed by touching the bones of the saint were really healed by thinking in a Certain Way, not by any power emanating from the relics. There is no healing power in the bones of dead people, whether they are those of saint or sinner.

✳ The people who were healed by the doses of either the allopath or the homeopath were also really healed by thinking in a Certain Way. There is no drug which has within itself the power to heal disease.

✳ The people who have been healed by prayers and affirmations were also healed by thinking in a Certain Way. There is no curative power in strings of words.

> *The two essentials of the Certain Way are:*
> *1) Faith, and*
> *2) the Personal Application of the Faith.*

The people who touched the saint's bones had faith. And so great was their faith that in the instant they touched the relics, they *severed all mental relations with disease, and mentally unified themselves with all health.*

This change of mind was accompanied by an intense devotional FEELING which penetrated to the deepest recesses of their souls, and so aroused the *Principle of Health* to powerful action. By faith, they claimed that they were healed, or appropriated health to themselves. In full faith, they ceased to think of themselves in connection with disease... and thought of themselves *only* in connection with health.

That which we make ourselves, mentally, we become physically; and that with which we unite ourselves mentally, we become unified with physically. If your thought always relates you to disease, then your thought becomes a fixed power to cause disease within you; and if your thought always relates you to health, then your thought becomes a fixed power exerted to keep you well.

In the case of the people who are healed by medicines, the result is obtained in the same way. They have, consciously or unconsciously, sufficient faith in the means used to cause them to sever mental relations with disease and to enter into mental relations with health.

Faith may be unconscious. It is possible for us to have an inner-conscious or inbred faith in things like medicine, in which we do not believe to any extent objectively; and yet, this inner-conscious faith may be quite sufficient to quicken the *Principle of Health* into constructive activity. Many who have little conscious faith are healed in this way; while many others who have great faith in the means are not healed because they do not make the *personal application to themselves.* Their faith is general, but not specific for their own case. A well-defined faith is easier to direct... and more effective as a result.

SUMMARY

The two essentials to thinking in the Certain Way, which will make you well are: first, claim or appropriate health by faith; and, second, sever all mental relations with disease, and enter into mental relations with healthfulness.

If you would consciously relate yourself to the All-Health, your purpose must be to live fully on every plane of your being. You must want all that there is in life for body, mind, and soul; and this will bring you into harmony with all the life there is. The person who is in conscious and intelligent harmony with All, will receive a continuous inflow of vital power from the Supreme Life; and this inflow is prevented by angry, selfish, or antagonistic mental attitudes. If you are against any part, you have severed relations with All; you will receive life, but only instinctively and automatically... not intelligently and purposefully. Be reconciled to everyone and everything.

In *The Science of Well-Being*, we have two main points to consider: how to think *with* faith; and how to so apply the thought to ourselves as to *quicken* the *Principle of Health* into constructive activity. We begin by learning what to think to become well.

CHAPTER FOUR

THINK YOURSELF WELL

*I*n order to sever all mental relations with disease, you must enter into mental relations with health, making the process positive not negative; one of assumption, not of rejection. *You are to receive or appropriate health, rather than to reject and deny disease! Denying disease accomplishes next to nothing.* It does little good to cast out the devil and leave the house vacant, for you will presently

> *You are to receive or appropriate health, rather than to reject and deny disease. Denying disease accomplishes next to nothing.*

return with others worse than himself. When you enter into the full and constant mental relations with health you must, out of necessity, cease all relationship with disease.

STEP 1: The first step in *The Science of Well-Being* is, then, to enter into complete thought-connection with health.

The best way to do this is to form a mental image or picture of yourself as being well, imagining a perfectly strong and healthy body. Spend sufficient time in contemplating this image to make it your habitual thought of yourself. Fortify your body with well-being by first believing and accepting healthfulness as a natural thought and way-of-life.

Imaging is not as easy as it sounds. It necessitates taking considerable time for meditation. Not all individuals have a well-developed imaging faculty, enough to form a distinct mental picture of themselves in a perfect or idealized body. It is much easier, as in *The Science of Getting Rich*, to form a mental image of the things we want to have; for we have seen these things, or their counterparts, in our surrounding material environment. We know how they look. We can picture them very easily from memory. But perhaps we have never seen ourselves in a perfect body, and a clear mental image is difficult to formulate, especially when it is so closely related to the physical self.

> *It is not necessary or essential, however, to have a clear mental image of yourself as you wish to be; it is only essential to form a CONCEPTION of perfect health, and to relate yourself to it.*

It is not necessary or essential, however, to have a clear mental image of yourself as you wish to be; it is only essential to form a CONCEPTION of perfect health, and to relate yourself to it. This Conception of Health is not a mental picture of a particular thing — it is an *understanding of health; an intention toward health,* and carries with it the idea of perfect functioning in every part and organ of the body.

45

> *Make yourself the central figure in the mental picture, doing things in an energetic, strong way.*

You may picture yourself as perfect in physique (cut a picture from a magazine of someone who exudes health, or get a past photo of yourself when you where "the picture of health"); this image will help you. And you MUST think of yourself as doing everything in the manner of a perfectly strong and healthy person. You can picture yourself as walking down the street with an erect body and a vigorous stride; you can picture yourself as doing your day's work easily and with surplus vigor, never tired or weak; you can picture in your mind how all things would be done by a person full of health and power. *Make yourself the central figure in the mental picture, doing things in an energetic, strong way.*

Never think of the ways in which weak or sickly people do things; always think of the way strong people do things. Spend your leisure time in thinking about the Strong Way, until you have a good conception of it; and always think of yourself in connection with the Strong Way of Doing

Things. This image is what we mean by having a *Conception of Health.*

In order to establish perfect functioning in every part of your body, you do not have to study anatomy or physiology. It is not necessary to form a mental image of each separate organ and address yourself to it. You do not have to "treat" your liver, your kidneys, your stomach, or your heart. There is ONE *Principle of Health* in you, which has control over all the involuntary functions of your life. The thought of perfect health, impressed upon this Principle, will reach each part and organ. Your liver is not controlled by a liver-principle, your stomach by a digestive-principle, and so on — the *Principle of Health* is ONE! — and Its reach is complete and wholistic in nature!

The less you go into the detailed study of physiology, the better for you. Human knowledge of this science is very imperfect, and leads to im-

> *The less you go into the detailed study of physiology, the better for you. Human knowledge of this science is very imperfect, and leads to imperfect thought. Imperfect thought causes imperfect functioning, which is disease.*

perfect thought. Imperfect thought causes imperfect functioning, which is disease. Let us illustrate: Until recently, physiology fixed ten days as the extreme limit of a human being's endurance without food; it was considered that only in exceptional cases could we survive a longer fast. So the impression became universally disseminated that a person who was deprived of food must die in from five to ten days. A numerous amount of people, when cut off from food by shipwreck, accident or famine, did die within this period.

The performances of fasting advocates, the writings on the fasting cure, and the experiments of numerous people who have fasted from forty to sixty days, show our ability to live without food is vastly greater than had been supposed. Any person, *properly educated*, can fast from twenty to forty days with little loss in weight, and often with no apparent loss of strength at all. The people who starved to death in ten days or less did so because they *believed* death was inevitable; an erroneous theory had given them a wrong thought about themselves. When a person is deprived of food they will die in from ten to fifty days, according to the way we have been taught; or, in other words, according to the way we think about starvation. So you see, an erroneous physiology can work very mischievous results.

No *Science of Well-Being* can be founded on current physiology; it is not sufficiently exact in its knowledge. With all its pretensions and preconceived notions, comparatively little is truly known about the interior workings and processes of the body and brain. It is not truly known just how food is digested; little is known of *exactly* what the liver, spleen, and pancreas are for, or what total part their secretions play in the chemistry of assimilation. Regarding these bodily functions and organs, we are able to theorize, yet to know concretely is merely an abstraction.

When you begin to study physiology, you enter the domain of theory and disputation; you come among conflicting opinions, and you are bound to form mistaken ideas concerning yourself. These mistaken ideas lead to the thinking of wrong thoughts, and this leads to perverted functioning and disease. We will show you the common-sense basics — how to eat, drink, breath, and sleep in a perfectly healthy way. This knowledge, as we have discussed earlier, lies within Original Substance, and can be accessed and acted upon — without studying physiology at all.

> *You cannot study any "science" which recognizes disease, if you are to think nothing but health.*

This idea, for the most part, is true of all hygiene. There are certain fundamental propositions which we should know; and these will be explained in later chapters. Aside from these propositions, *ignore physiology and hygiene* – they tend to fill your mind with thoughts of imperfect conditions, and these thoughts will produce the imperfect conditions in your own body. *You cannot study any "science" which recognizes disease, if you are to think nothing but health.* A healthful you will result with thought and concentration on the state of well-being. It is only YOU who can command your own thoughts!

✳ Drop all investigation as to your present condition, its causes, or possible results, and set yourself to the work of forming a *Conception of Health.*

✳ Think about health and the possibilities of health; of the work which may be done, and the pleasures which may be enjoyed in a condition of perfect health. Make this conception your guide in thinking of yourself. Refuse to entertain, for an instant, any thought of yourself which is not in harmony with perfect wellness. When any thought of disease or imperfect functioning enters your mind, cast it out instantly by calling up a thought which is in harmony with the *Conception of Health.*

✳ Think of yourself at all times as realizing conception; as being a strong and perfectly healthy individual. Do not harbor a contrary thought.

✳ Know that as you think of yourself in unity with this conception, the Original Substance which permeates and fills the tissues of your body is taking form according to your thought.

✳ Know that this Intelligent Substance or Mind-Stuff will cause function to be performed in such a way that your body will be rebuilt with perfectly healthy cells.

The Intelligent Substance, from which all things are made, permeates and penetrates all things; and so It is in and through your body. It moves according to Its thoughts. So, if you hold only the thoughts of perfectly healthy function, It will cause the movements of perfectly healthy function within you.

✳ Hold with persistence to the thought of perfect health in relation to yourself; do not permit yourself to think in any other way. Hold this thought with perfect faith that it is in fact, the truth. It is the truth so far as your mental body is concerned.

✳ Eliminate reading books, articles, or advertisements, and viewing television shows, and commercials which depict disease, death, and destruction. They will only fill your mind with pictures contrary to the Conception of Health.

You have a mind-body and a physical-body. The mind-body takes form just as you think of yourself, and any thought which you hold continuously is made visible by the transformation of the physical-body into its image. Implanting the thought of perfect functioning in the mind-body will, in due time, cause perfect functioning in the physical-body.

> In the creation and recreation of forms, Substance moves along the fixed lines of growth It has established; and the impression upon It of the health-thought causes the healthy body to be built cell by cell.

The transformation of the physical-body into the image of the ideal held by the mind-body is not accomplished instantaneously (we cannot transfigure our physical bodies at will, as Jesus did... not yet). In the creation and recreation of forms, *Substance moves along the fixed lines of growth It has established;* and the impression upon It of the health-thought causes the healthy body to be built cell by cell. Holding only thoughts of perfect health will ultimately cause perfect functioning; and perfect functioning will, in due time, produce a perfectly healthy body.

SUMMARY

Your physical-body is permeated and filled with an Intelligent Substance, which forms a body of Mind-Stuff. This Mind-Stuff controls the functioning of your physical-body. A thought of disease or of imperfect function, impressed upon the Mind-Stuff, causes disease or imperfect functioning in the physical-body. If you are diseased, it is because wrong thoughts have made impressions on this Mind-Stuff; these may have been either your own thoughts, or those of your parents or of your environment. We begin life with many inner-conscious impressions, both right and wrong. But the natural tendency of All-Mind is toward health, and if no thoughts are held in the conscious mind except those of health, all internal functioning will come to be performed in a perfectly healthy manner.

The Power of Nature within you is sufficient to overcome all hereditary impressions. If you will learn to control your thoughts, so that you will focus your thoughts only on those of healthfulness, and if you will perform the voluntary functions of life in a perfectly healthy way, you certainly can be well.

CHAPTER FIVE

BELIEVE YOURSELF WELL

*T*he *Principle of Health* is moved by Faith or Belief; nothing else can call it into action, and only faith can enable you to relate yourself to health, and sever your relation with disease.

You will continue to think of disease unless you have faith in well-being. If you do not have faith, you will doubt; if you doubt, you will fear; and if you fear, you will relate your mind-set to that which you fear.

> *You will continue to think of disease unless you have faith in well-being. If you do not have faith you will doubt; if you doubt, you will fear; and if you fear, you will relate your mind-set to that which you fear.*

As a result of fear, many of us go through life, if not actually diseased, in the constant fear that this form of sickness or that will come upon us, until we become a constant burden to ourselves and others. As the old Oriental proverb puts it: "The plague killed five thousand people. Fifty thousand died of fear."

If you fear disease, you will think of yourself in connection with disease, which will produce within yourself the form and motions of disease. Just as Original Substance creates from Itself the forms of Its thoughts, so your mind-body, which *is* Original Substance, takes the form and motion of whatever you think about. If you fear disease, dread disease, have doubts about your safety from disease, or if you even contemplate disease — you will connect yourself with it and create its forms and motions within yourself. *Avoid disease by separating your thoughts from it!*

Let us enlarge somewhat upon this point. The potency, or creative power, of a thought is given to it by the faith placed in it.

> THOUGHTS WHICH CONTAIN NO FAITH CREATE NO FORMS.

The Formless Substance, which knows all truth and therefore thinks only truth, has perfect faith in every thought. Because It thinks only truth; all of Its thoughts create and effect action.

But if you will imagine a thought in Formless Substance devoid of faith, you will see that such a thought could not cause Substance to move or take form.

Keep in mind the fact that *only those thoughts which are conceived in faith have creative energy. Only those thoughts which have faith with them are able to change function, or to quicken the Principle of Health into activity.*

> ✳ If you do not have faith in health, you will certainly have faith in disease.
>
> ✳ If you do not have faith in health, it will do you no good to think about health, for your thoughts will have no potency,

and will cause no change for the better in your condition.

✳ If you do not have faith in health, we repeat, you will have faith in disease; and if, under such conditions, you think about health for ten hours a day, and think about disease for only a few minutes, the disease-thought will still control your condition because it will have the potency of faith, while the health-thought will not. Your mind-body will take on the form and motions of disease and retain them, because your health-thought will not have sufficient dynamic force to change form or motion.

In order to practice *The Science of Well-Being*, you must have complete faith in healthfulness.

Faith begins in belief; therefore, we now come to the question: What must you believe in order to have faith in your health?

You must believe there is more health-power than disease-power in both yourself and your environment. You cannot help but believe in this if you consider these facts:

✳ *FACT:* There is a Thinking Substance from which all things are made, and which, in its original state, permeates, penetrates, and fills the interspaces of the Universe.

✳ *FACT:* The thought of a form, in this Substance, produces the form; the thought of a motion institutes the motion. In relation to humans, the thoughts of Original Substance are always of perfect health and perfect functioning. This Substance, within and without us, always exerts Its power toward health.

✳ *FACT:* You are a thinking center, capable of original thought. You have a mind-body of Original Substance permeating a physical-body; and the functioning of your physical-body is determined by the FAITH of your mind-body. If you think, with complete faith, of health, you will cause your internal organs to perform in a healthy manner (provided you perform the external functions in a corresponding healthy manner). But if you think, with faith, of disease, or of the power of disease, you will cause your internal functioning to be disease-ridden.

✳ *FACT:* The Original Intelligent Substance is in you, moving toward health; and It is pressing upon you from every side. You live, move, and have your being in a limitless ocean of health-power; and you use this power according to your faith. If you appropriate it, and apply it to yourself, It is all yours; and if you unify yourself with It by unquestioning faith, you cannot fail to attain health. The power of this Substance is all the power there is and with faith, well-being is all-existent.

Belief in the above statements is a foundation for faith in health. If you believe them 1) you believe health is the natural state of humans, and you live in the midst of Universal Health; all the power of nature makes for healthfulness, and health is possible to all, and can surely be attained by all. 2) You will believe the power of health in the universe is ten-thousand-times greater than that of disease — in fact, disease has no power whatever, being only the result of perverted thought and faith. 3) And if you believe health is possible to you, and that it may surely be attained by you, and you know exactly what to do in order to attain it, you will have faith in health. You will have this faith and knowledge if you read this book through with care, and determine to believe in and practice its teachings.

It is not merely the possession of faith, but the PERSONAL APPLICATION OF FAITH which works the healing.

STEP 1: You must claim health in the beginning, and form a Conception of Health of yourself as a perfectly healthy person.

STEP 2: Then, by faith, you must claim you ARE REALIZING this conception.

Do not assert with faith that you are going to get well; assert with faith that you ARE well. Having faith in health, and applying it to yourself, means having the belief you are healthy; and the *first step in this process is to claim that it is the truth.*

Mentally take the attitude of well-being, and do not say anything or do anything which contradicts this attitude. Never speak a word or assume a physical attitude which does not harmonize with the claim: "I am perfectly well." When you walk, go with a brisk step, and with your shoulders back and your head held up. Watch at all times that your physical actions and attitudes are those of a healthy person. When you find yourself relapsing into the attitude of weakness or disease, change instantly — straighten up; think of health and power. Refuse to consider yourself as other than a perfectly healthy person.

One great aid — perhaps the greatest one — in applying your faith, you will find in the exercise of GRATITUDE: *Whenever you think of yourself, or of your advancing condition, give thanks to the Great Intelligent Substance for the perfect health you are enjoying.*

Remember, there is a continual inflow of life from the Supreme, which is received by all created things according to their forms; and by the person according to their faith. Health from God is continually being urged upon you. When you think of this, lift up your mind reverently to Him, and give thanks that you have been led to the Truth and into perfect health of mind and body. Be, all the time, in a grateful frame of mind, and let gratitude be evident in your speech.

> *GRATITUDE WILL HELP YOU TO OWN AND CONTROL YOUR OWN FIELD-OF-THOUGHT.*

Whenever the thought of disease is presented to you, instantly claim health, and thank the Infinite for the perfect health you have. Do this act so there will be no room in your mind for a thought of illness. Your every thought connected in any way with ill-health is unwelcome. You can close the door of your mind in its face by asserting you are well, and by reverently thanking the Source that this state of wellness is true. Soon the old thoughts of disease and sickness no longer return.

> Gratitude has a two-fold effect:
> ✳ 1) it strengthens your own faith, and
> ✳ 2) it brings you into close and harmonious relations with the Supreme.

The ungrateful or unthankful mind really denies that it receives at all, and so cuts its connection with the Supreme. The grateful mind is always looking toward the Supreme, and is always open to receive from It; and the grateful mind will receive continually.

SUMMARY

You believe there is one Intelligent Substance from which all life and all power come; you believe that you receive your own life from this Substance; and you relate yourself closely to It by feeling continuous gratitude. It is easy to see the more closely you relate yourself to the Source of Life, the more readily you may receive life from It; and it is easy also to *see your relation to It is a matter of mental attitude.*

We cannot come into *physical* relationship with God, for God is mind-stuff, and we also are mind-stuff; our relation with Him must therefore be a *mind relationship.* It is plain, then, that the person who feels deep and hearty gratitude will live in closer touch with the Supreme than the person who never looks to Him in thankfulness.

The *Principle of Health* in you receives its vital power from the Principle of Life in the Universe; and you relate yourself to the Principle of Life by faith in health, and by gratitude for the health you receive. *You may cultivate both faith and gratitude by the proper use of your will.*

CHAPTER SIX

WILL YOURSELF WELL

*I*n the practice of *The Science of Well-Being,* the will is not used to compel yourself to go when you are not truly able to go. It does not propel you to do things when you are not physically strong enough to do them. You do not direct your will upon your physical-body or try to compel the proper performance of internal function by will power.

> You direct your will upon the mind, and use it in determining what you will believe, what you will think, and to what you will give your attention.

You direct your will upon the mind, and use it in determining what you will believe, what you will think, and to what you will give your attention.

You should never use the will upon any person or thing external to you. It should never be used upon your own body. *The sole legitimate use of the will is in determining to what you will give your attention, and what you will think about the things to which your attention is given.* For example, in the light of health and unhealthiness, you should will your thoughts on healthiness. Then, and only after this step, can you will further thoughts on the state of well-being.

All belief begins in the will to believe. You cannot always and instantly believe what you will to believe; but you can always will to believe what you *want* to believe. If you want to believe thoughts about healthfulness, you can will yourself to do so. The statements you have been reading in this book are the truth about health, and you can will yourself to believe in them; this must be your first step toward getting well.

The following are statements you must will to believe:

✳ 1. That there is a Thinking Substance from which all things are made, and that you receive, the Principle of Health, which is your life, from this Substance.

✳ 2. That you yourself are Thinking Substance; mind-body, permeating a physical-body, and as your thoughts are, so will be the functioning of your physical-body. So... think healthy thoughts!

✳ 3. That if you will think only thoughts of perfect health, you must and will cause the internal and involuntary functioning of your body to be the functioning of health, provided that your external and voluntary functioning and attitude are in accordance with your thoughts.

When you *will* to believe these statements, you must also begin to act upon them:

* You cannot long *retain* a belief unless you act upon it.
* You cannot *increase* a belief until it becomes faith, and unless you act upon it.
* You cannot expect to *reap benefits* in any way from a belief so long as you act as if the opposite were true.

You cannot sustain or prolong faith in health if you continue to act like a sick person. If you continue to act like a sick person, you cannot help but to continue to think of yourself as a sick person; and if you continue to think of yourself as a sick person, you will continue to be a sick person.

The first step toward acting externally like a well person is to begin to act internally like a well person. Form your Conception of Perfect Health, and get into the way of thinking about perfect health until it begins to have a definite meaning to you. Picture yourself as doing the things a strong and healthy person would do, and have faith you can and will do those things in that way. Continue this mental image until you have a vivid CONCEPTION of Health, and what it means to you.

When we speak in this book of *Conception of Health*, we mean a conception that carries with it the idea of the way a healthy person looks and acts. Think of yourself in connection with health until you form a conception of how you would live, appear, act, and operate as a perfectly healthy person. Think about yourself in connection with health until you conceive of yourself, in imagination, as always doing everything in the manner of a well person; until the thought of health conveys the idea of what health means to you. As we have said in a former chapter, you may not be able to form a clear mental image of yourself in perfect health, but you can form a conception of yourself as acting like a healthy person. In this self-image, you should picture a completely healthy YOU — in mental, spiritual, and physical wellness.

Form this conception, and then think only thoughts of perfect health in relation to yourself, and (as much as possible) in relation to others. When a thought of sickness or disease is presented to you, reject it; do not let it get into your mind; do not entertain or consider it at all! Meet it by thinking health; by thinking that you are well, and by being sincerely grateful for the health you are receiving.

Guard your speech; make every word harmonize with the conception of perfect health. Never complain; never say things like: "I did not sleep well last night;" "I have a pain in my side"; "I do not feel at all well today," and so on. Say, "I am looking forward to a good night's sleep"; "I can see I am progressing rapidly," and things of similar meaning. In so far as everything which is connected with *disease* is concerned, your way is to forget it; and in so far as everything which is connected with *health* is concerned, your way is to unify yourself with it in thought and speech.

Relate not only yourself, but so far as possible all others, in your thoughts, to perfect health. Do not sympathize with people when they complain, or even when they are sick and suffering. Turn their thoughts into a constructive channel if you can; do all you can for their relief, but do it with the health-thought in your mind.

Do not let people tell their woes and catalog their symptoms to you; turn the conversation to some other subject, or excuse yourself and leave. Better be considered an unfeeling person than to have the disease-thought forced upon

> *No matter what they think or say; politeness does not require you to permit yourself to be poisoned by diseased or perverted thought.*

you. When you are in the company of people whose conversational stock-in-trade is sickness and like matters, ignore what they say and fall to offering a mental prayer of gratitude for your perfect health. And if that does not enable you to shut out their thoughts, say good-bye and leave them.

No matter what they think or say; politeness does not require you to permit yourself to be poisoned by diseased or perverted thought. When we have a few more hundreds of thousands of enlightened thinkers who will not stay where people complain and talk of sickness, the world will advance rapidly toward health. When you let people talk to you of sickness, you assist them to increase and multiply sickness.

Whenever suggestions of disease are coming thick and fast upon you, and you are in a "tight place," fall back upon the exercise of gratitude. Connect yourself with the Supreme; give thanks to God for the perfect health He gives you. You will soon find yourself able to control your thoughts, and to think what you want to think. In times of doubt, trial, and temptation — the exercise of gratitude is always a strong anchor which will prevent you from being swept away. Remember, the great essential thing is to...

> SEVER ALL MENTAL RELATIONS WITH DISEASE, AND ENTER INTO FULL MENTAL RELATIONSHIP WITH HEALTH.

This is the KEY to all mental healing; it is the cure to ALL! Here we see the secret of the great success of Christian Science; more than any other formulated system of practice, it insists that its converts will sever relations with disease, and relate themselves fully to health. The healing power of Christian Science is not in its theological formula, nor in its denial of matter; but in the fact that it induces the sick to ignore disease as an unreal thing and accept health by faith as a reality. Its failures are made because its practitioners, while thinking in the Certain Way, do not eat, drink, breathe, and sleep in the same way. Therefore, their external actions do not coordinate with their internal thoughts. Faith is not present and flowing. Sickness is, then, a result.

While there is no healing power in the repetition of strings of words, it is a very convenient thing to have the central thoughts so formulated you can repeat them readily; so you can use them as affirmations or *Alphamatics* (affirmations said in a meditative Alpha brain level), whenever you are surrounded by an environment which gives you adverse suggestions. When those around you begin to talk of sickness and death, close your ears and mentally assert something like the following:

There is One Substance, and I am that Substance.
That Substance is Eternal, and it is Life;
I am that Substance, and I am Eternal Life.
That Substance knows no disease;
I am that Substance, and I am Health.

Exercise your will power in choosing only those thoughts which are thoughts of health, and arrange your environment so it will suggest thoughts of health. In other words, if you surround yourself with internal and external health

— the natural consequence will be mental and physical health!

> ✳ Do not surround yourself with books, pictures, or other things which suggest death, disease, deformity, weakness, or age; have only those which convey the ideas of health, power, joy, vitality, and youth!

Do not read "doctor books" or medical literature, or the literature of those whose theories conflict with those set forth here. To do so will certainly undermine your faith in the Way of Living upon which you have entered, and cause you to again come into mental relations with disease. This book truly gives you all that is required; nothing essential has been omitted, and practically all the superfluous has been eliminated. *The Science of Well-Being* is an exact science, like arithmetic; nothing can be added to the fundamental principles, and if anything can be taken from them, an error will result. *You must think only health, recognize only health, and give your attention only to health; and you must control thought, recognition, and attention by the use of your will.*

✳ Do not try to use your will to compel healthy performance of function within you. The *Principle of Health* will attend to that, if you give your attention only to thoughts of health.

> *... you must think only health, recognize only health, and give your attention only to health; and you must control thought, recognition, and attention by the use of your will.*

✳ Do not try to exert your will upon the Formless to compel It to give you more vitality or power; It is already placing all the power there is at your service.

✳ Do not use your will to conquer adverse conditions, or to subdue unfriendly forces; there are no unfriendly forces; there is only One Force, and that force is friendly to you; It is a force which makes for health.

Q. What will I do when I am in pain? Can I be in actual physical suffering and still think only thoughts of health?

A. Yes. Do not resist pain; recognize it is a good thing. Pain is caused by an effort of the *Principle of Health* to overcome some unnatural condition; this you must know and feel.

When you have a pain, think that a process of healing is going on in the affected part, and mentally assist and cooperate with it. Put yourself in full mental harmony with the Power which is causing the pain; assist it; help it along. Do not hesitate, when necessary, to use hot liquids and ointments, and similar means to further the good work which is going on.

If the pain is severe, lie down and give your mind to the work of quietly and easily co-operating with the Force which is at work for your good. This is the time to exercise gratitude and faith. Be thankful for the Power of Health which is causing the pain, and be certain the pain will cease as soon as the good work is done. Fix your thoughts, with confidence, on the *Principle of Health* which is working within to eliminate the conditions of unnecessary pain. You will be surprised to find how easily you can conquer pain; and after you have lived for a time in this Scientific Way, aches and pains will be unknown to you.

Q. What will I do when I am too weak for my work? Shall I drive myself beyond my strength; trusting in the Infinite to support me? Shall I go on, like the runner, expecting a "second wind"?

A. No; better not. When you begin to live in this Way, you will not be of normal strength; and using these methods, you will gradually pass from a low physical condition to a higher one. If you relate yourself mentally with health and strength, and perform the voluntary functions of life in a perfectly healthy manner, your strength will increase from day to day. However, for a time you may have days when your strength is insufficient for the work you would like to do. At such times rest, and exercise gratitude. Recognize the fact that your strength is growing rapidly, and feel a deep thankfulness to the Living One from whom it comes. Spend an hour of weakness in thanksgiving and rest, with full faith that great strength is at hand; and then get up and go on again. While you rest, do not think of your present weakness; think of the strength that is coming.

Never, at any time, allow yourself to think you are giving way to weakness. When you rest, as when you go to sleep, fix your mind on the *Principle of Health* which is building you into complete strength.

SUMMARY

Everything in the Universe wants you to be well; you have absolutely nothing to overcome but your own habit of thinking in a certain way about disease, and you can do this only by forming a habit of thinking in another Certain Way about health.

You can cause all the internal functions of your body to be performed in a perfectly healthy manner by continuously thinking in a Certain Way, and by performing the external functions in a Certain Way.

You can think in this Certain Way by controlling your attention, and you can control your attention by the use of your will.

You can and MUST decide what things you will think about!

CHAPTER SEVEN

HEALTH FROM THE SUPREME

*W*hat do we mean by the *Supreme?* By the Supreme we mean the Thinking Substance from which all things are made, and which is in all and through all, seeking more complete expression and fuller life.

This Intelligent Substance, in a perfectly fluid state, permeates and penetrates all things, and is in touch with all minds. It is the source of all energy and power, and constitutes the "inflow" of life which vitalizes all things. It is working to one

definite end, and for the fulfillment of one purpose; and *this purpose is the advancement of life
toward the complete expression of Mind.* When you
harmonize yourself with this Intelligence, It can
and will give you health and wisdom. When you
hold steadily to the purpose to live more abundantly, you come into harmony with this Supreme
Intelligence.

The purpose of the Supreme Intelligence is
the most Abundant Life for all; the purpose of this
Supreme Intelligence for you is that you should
live more abundantly. If, then, your own purpose
is to live more abundantly, you are unified with
the Supreme; you are working with It, and It must
work with you. But as the Supreme Intelligence is
in all, if you harmonize with It, you must harmonize with all; and you must desire more abundant
life for all, as well as for yourself. Two great benefits come to you from being in harmony with the
Supreme Intelligence.

> ✳ 1. *You will receive wisdom.* By wisdom
> we do not mean knowledge of facts so
> much as ability to perceive and under-
> stand facts, and to judge soundly and act
> rightly in all matters relating to life.

WISDOM is the power to perceive truth, and the ability to make the best use of the knowledge of truth. It is the power to perceive at once the best end to aim at, and the means best adapted to attain this end. With wisdom comes poise, and the power to think rightly; to control and guide your thoughts, and to avoid the difficulties which come from wrong thinking. With wisdom you will be able to select the right courses for your particular needs. You will then govern yourself in all ways as to secure the best results. You will know how to effect what you want to do.

You can readily see wisdom must be an essential attribute of the Supreme Intelligence, since That which knows all truth must be wise; and you can also see just in proportion as you harmonize and unify your mind with that Intelligence, you will have wisdom.

But we repeat, since this Intelligence is All, and in all, you can enter into Its wisdom only by harmonizing with all. If there is anything in your desire or your purpose which will bring oppression to any, or bring injustice to, or cause lack of life for any, you cannot receive wisdom from the Supreme. Furthermore, your purpose for your own self must be the best.

> Wisdom is the power to perceive truth, and the ability to make the best use of the knowledge of truth. It is the power to perceive at once the best end to aim at, and the means best adapted to attain that end.

You are recommended to read what we have said in a former work *The Science of Getting Rich* concerning the *competitive mind* and the *creative mind*. It is very doubtful whether one who has lost health can completely regain it so long as they remain in the competitive mind. Want for every person all that you want for yourself.

You can live in three general ways: for the gratification 1) of your body; 2) for your intellect; or 3) for your soul. The first is accomplished by satisfying the desires for food, drink, and those other things which give enjoyable physical sensations. The second is accomplished by doing those things which cause pleasant mental sensations, such as gratifying the desire for knowledge or those for fine clothing, fame, power, and so on. The third is accomplished by giving way to the instincts of unselfish love and altruism. *You live most wisely and completely when you function most perfectly along all of these lines, without excess in any of them.*

The person who lives selfishly, for the body alone, is unwise and out of harmony with Source; the person who lives solely for the cold enjoyments of the intellect, though he or she be absolutely moral, is unwise and out of harmony with Source; and the person who lives wholly for the practice of altruism, and who throws himself or herself away for others, is as unwise and as far from harmony with Source as those who go to excess in other ways.

To come into full harmony with the Supreme, you must purpose to LIVE; to live to the utmost of your capabilities in body, mind, and soul. This must mean the full exercise of function in all the different ways, but without excess; for *excess in one causes deficiency in the others*. Behind your desire for health is your own desire for more abundant life; and behind that is the desire of the Formless Intelligence to live more fully in you. So, as you advance toward perfect health, hold steadily to the purpose to attain complete life — physical, mental, and spiritual; to advance in all ways, and in every way to live more. If you hold to this purpose, you will be given wisdom. "He who wills to do the will of the Father will KNOW," said Jesus. *Wisdom is the most desirable gift that can come to you, for it makes you rightly self-governing.*

> ✳ 2. But wisdom is not all you may receive from the Supreme Intelligence. *You may receive physical energy, vitality, and life force.* The energy of the Formless Substance is unlimited, and permeates everything.

You are already receiving or appropriating to yourself this energy in an automatic and instinctive way. But you can do so to a far greater degree if you set about it intelligently. The measure of your strength is not what God is willing to give you, but whether you, yourself, have the will and the intelligence to appropriate it yourself. God gives you all there is; your only question is how much to take of the *unlimited* supply.

There is apparently no limit to the powers of humans; and this bounty is simply because our power comes from the inexhaustible reservoir of the Supreme. The runner who has reached the stage of exhaustion, when his or her physical power seems entirely gone, can continue by running on in a Certain Way, and receive his or her "second wind"; their strength is renewed in a seemingly miraculous fashion, and they can go on indefinitely. And by continuing in the Certain Way, they may receive a third, fourth, and fifth "wind"; we do not know where the limit is, or how far it may be possible to extend it. The conditions are that the runner must have absolute faith the strength will come. In the same light, you must think steadily of strength, and have perfect confidence that you have it, and you must continue to run on. If you admit a doubt into your mind, you fall exhausted. If you stop running to wait for the accession of strength, it will never come. Put your faith in strength; your faith that you can keep on running; your unwavering purpose to keep on running, and your action in keeping on will connect you to the Source of Energy in such a way as to bring you a new supply.

In a very similar manner, the sick person who has unquestioning faith in health, whose purpose brings them into harmony with the Source, and who performs the voluntary functions of life in a Certain Way, will receive vital energy sufficient for all their needs, and for the healing of all their diseases.

SUMMARY

The Creative Source, who seeks to live and express Himself fully in us, delights to give us all which is needed for the most abundant life. Action and reaction are equal, and when you desire to live more, if you are in mental harmony with the Supreme, the forces which make for life begin to concentrate about you and upon you. The One Life begins to move toward you, and your environment becomes surcharged with it. Then, if you appropriate it by faith, it is yours. "Ye will ask what ye will, and it will be done unto you." Your Father gives not His spirit by measure; He delights to give good gifts to you.

PART II

EAT TO ENJOY GOOD HEALTH

CHAPTER EIGHT

WHEN TO EAT

*Y*ou cannot build and maintain a perfectly healthy body by mental action alone, or by the performance of the inner-conscious or involuntary functions alone. There are certain actions, more or less *voluntary*, which have a direct and immediate relation with the continuance of life itself — these are eating, drinking, breathing, and sleeping. No matter what your thought or mental attitude may be, you cannot live unless you eat, drink, breathe, and sleep. Moreover, you cannot be well if you eat, drink, breathe, and sleep in an unnatural or unfit manner. It is therefore vitally important that you should learn the right way to perform these voluntary functions. We will proceed to show you this way, beginning with one of the most important matters — eating.

There has been a vast amount of controversy as to when to eat, what to eat, how to eat, and how much to eat. All this controversy is unnecessary, for the Right Way is very easy to find. You have only to consider the Law which governs all attainment, whether of health, wealth, power, or happiness.

> ✳ *LAW:* You must do what you can do now, where you are now; do every separate act in the most perfect manner possible, and put the power of faith into every action.

The processes of digestion and assimilation are under the supervision and control of an inner division of our mentality, which is generally called the *inner-conscious mind* (we will use that term here in order to be understood). The inner-conscious mind is in charge of all the functions and processes of life. For example, when more food is needed by the body, it makes the fact known by causing a sensation called hunger. Whenever food is needed, and can be used, there is hunger; and whenever there is hunger, it is time to eat. When there is no hunger it is unnatural and wrong to eat — no matter how great the need for food may APPEAR to be. Even if you are in a condition of apparent starvation, with great emaciation, if there is no hunger, you may know that FOOD CANNOT BE USED. It will be unnatural and improper for you to eat. Though you have not eaten for days, weeks, or months, if you have no hunger you may be perfectly sure food cannot be used, and will probably not be used if taken.

Whenever food is needed, if there is power to digest and assimilate it, so that it can be normally used, the inner-conscious mind will announce the fact by a decided hunger. Food, taken when there is no hunger, will sometimes be digested and assimilated, because Nature makes a special effort to perform the task which is thrust upon Her against Her will. However, if food is habitually taken when there is no hunger, the digestive power is at last destroyed, and numerous ills are a result.

> ALWAYS *eat when you are hungry; and NEVER eat when you are not hungry. This is obedience to nature, which is obedience to the Source.*

If the foregoing be true — and it is indisputably so — it is a self-evident proposition that the natural time, and the healthy time, to eat is when one is hungry; and it is never a natural or a healthy action to eat when one is not hungry. You see, then, it is an easy matter to scientifically settle the question when to eat. *ALWAYS eat when you are hungry; and NEVER eat when you are not hungry. This is obedience to nature, which is obedience to the Source.*

You must not fail, however, to make clear the distinction between hunger and appetite.

> *HUNGER* is the call of the inner-conscious mind for more material to be used in repairing and renewing the body, and in keeping up the internal heat. Hunger is never felt unless there is need for more material, and unless there is power to digest it when taken into the stomach.

APPETITE is a desire for the gratification of sensation. The alcoholic has an appetite for liquor, but they cannot have a hunger for it. A normally fed person cannot have a hunger for candy or sweets; the desire for these things is an appetite. You cannot hunger for tea, coffee, spiced foods, or for the various taste-tempting dishes of the skilled cook; if you desire these things, it is with appetite, not with hunger. *Hunger is Nature's call for material to be used in building new cells, and Nature never calls for anything which may not be legitimately used for this purpose.*

Appetite is often largely a matter of habit: if one eats or drinks at a certain hour, and especially if one takes sweetened, or spicy and stimulating foods, the desire comes regularly at the same hour. This habitual desire for food should never be mistaken for hunger. Hunger does not appear at specified times. It only comes when work or exercise has destroyed sufficient tissue to make the taking in of new material a necessity. Remember, a healthy hunger is a result of healthy activity.

> *No matter who you are, or what your condition; no matter how hard you work, or how much you are exposed... unless you go to your bed starved, you cannot arise from your bed hungry.*

Appetite is a product of habit and perception. To reach a state of well-being in eating means to satisfy hunger, not appetite!

For instance, if you have sufficiently eaten on the preceding day, it is impossible that you should feel a genuine hunger upon awakening from a refreshing sleep. In sleep, the body is recharged with vital power, and the assimilation of the food eaten during the day is completed. Your system has no need for food immediately after sleep, unless you went to bed in a state of starvation.

With a system of eating (which is even a reasonable approach to a natural one), *no one can have a real hunger for an early morning breakfast.* There is no such physical possibility as a normal or genuine hunger immediately after arising from sound sleep. The early morning breakfast is always taken to gratify appetite, never to satisfy hunger. This appetite is more a state-of-mind rather than a healthy state-of-being. No matter who you are, or what your condition; no matter how hard you work, or how much you are exposed... unless you go to your bed starved, you cannot arise from your bed hungry.

Q. But if I do not eat on arising in the morning, when will I eat my first meal?

A. In ninety-nine cases out of a hundred, twelve o'clock, noon, is early enough (approximately four hours after rising if you sleep at varied times); and it is generally the most convenient time. If you are doing heavy work, you will reach noon time with a hunger sufficient to justify a good-sized meal; and if your work is light, you will probably still have hunger enough for a moderate meal. The best general rule or law that can be laid down is you should eat your first meal of the day at noon, provided you are hungry; and provided you are not hungry, wait until you become so.

Q. And when will I eat my second meal?

A. Not at all, unless you are hungry for it; and that with a genuine earned hunger. If you do get hungry for a second meal, eat at the most convenient time; but do not eat until you have an over-whelming hunger. If you surpass the line of earned hunger into starvation — your eating will become unnatural and unhealthy.

Q. Are long continued fasts necessary?

A. Seldom, if ever. The *Principle of Health* does not often require twenty, thirty, or forty days to get ready for action; under normal conditions, hunger will come in much less time. In most long fasts, the reason hunger does not come sooner is because it has been inhibited by the patient themselves. They begin the fast with the FEAR, if not actually with the hope, that it will be many days before hunger comes. The literature they have read on the subject has prepared them to expect a long fast, and they are doggedly determined to go to a finish, let the time be as long as it will. And the inner-conscious mind, under the influence of powerful and positive suggestion, suspends hunger.

Fasting (medically supervised) is the only remedy, in some cases, that will permit the body system to throw off disease, and come to a *physiological equilibrium*, but it is a mistaken idea that fasting cures disease. The cure is to come after the fast, for the disease was brought on by wrong living, and fasting will not cure errors of life any more than any other so-called cure.

When, for any reason, Nature takes away your hunger, go cheerfully on with your usual work, and do not eat until She gives it back. No matter if it is two, three, ten days, or longer; you may be perfectly sure that when it is time for you to eat, you will be hungry. And if you are cheerfully confident and keep your faith in health, you will suffer from no weakness or discomfort caused by abstinence. When you are not hungry, you will feel stronger, happier, and more comfortable if you do not eat, than you will if you do eat; no matter how long the fast. And if you live in the Scientific Way described in this book, you will never have to take long fasts; you will seldom miss a meal, and you will enjoy your meals more than ever before in your life. Get an earned hunger before you eat; and whenever you get an earned hunger... eat!

SUMMARY

You cannot think perfect health so long as you know you are living in a wrong or unhealthy way; or even so long as you have doubts, or are confused, as to whether or not you are living in a healthy way. You must not only think of yourself as perfectly healthy, but you must also perform the voluntary functions of eating, breathing, and sleeping in a perfectly healthy manner.

In eating, you must learn to be guided by your hunger. You must distinguish between hunger and appetite, and between hunger and the cravings of habit. Genuine hunger is never present after natural sleep. *Hunger is not caused by sleep, but by work!* And it does not matter who you are, or what your condition, or how hard or easy your work. The so-called "no-breakfast plan" is the right plan for you. *It is the right plan for everyone, because it is based on the Universal Law that hunger never comes until it is EARNED. Sleep revitalizes your energy... it does not detract from it.*

We are aware that protests against this may come from the large number of people who "enjoy" their breakfasts; from those who claim breakfast is their "best meal"; who believe their work is so hard that they cannot "get through the morning on an empty stomach." But all their arguments fall apart before the facts. They enjoy their breakfast as the alcoholic enjoys a morning drink, because it gratifies a habitual appetite and not because it supplies a natural want! It is their best meal for the same reason that the morning dram is the alcoholic's best drink... and which they CAN get along without! Millions of people, of every trade and profession, DO get along without breakfast, and are vastly better for doing so. If you are to live according to *The Science of Well-Being*, you must NEVER EAT UNTIL YOU HAVE AN EARNED HUNGER!

(For further information, read the books mentioned in the *Preface*.) From the foregoing, however, you can easily see that *The Science of Well-Being* readily answers the question: When, and how often will I eat? The answer is:

> *Eat when you have an earned hunger; and never eat at any other time.*

CHAPTER NINE

WHAT TO EAT

*T*he current sciences of medicine and hygiene have made no progress toward answering the question, "What will I eat?" The contests between the vegetarians and the meat-eaters, the cooked-food advocates, raw-food advocates, and various other "schools" of theorists, seem to be interminable. There exists mountains of evidence and argument piled up for and against each special theory. However, it is plain to see, if we depend on these scientists, we will never know (or run in circles trying to discover!) what is the natural food for humans. Turning away from the whole controversy, we will ask the question of Nature herself, to find she has not left us without an answer.

Most of the errors of dietary scientists grow out of a false premise as to the natural state of human beings. It is assumed that civilization and mental development are unnatural things: that the person who lives in a modern house, in city or country, and who works in modern trade or industry for his or her living is leading an unnatural life, and is in an unnatural environment; that the only "natural" person is a naked savage, and that the farther we get from the savage, the farther we are from nature. This is wrong! You, who have all the benefits which art and science can give, are leading the most natural life. Why? Because you are living most completely in all your faculties. The tenant in a well-appointed city apartment, with modern conveniences and good ventilation, is living a far more naturally human life than the Australian aborigine who lives in a hollow tree or a hole in the ground.

That Great Intelligence, which is in all and through all, has in reality, practically settled the question as to what we will eat. In ordering the affairs of Nature, It decided what and where the most necessary foods humans would require, according to the zone of habitat. In the frigid regions of the FAR NORTH, fuel foods are required. Life is not severe in its labor-tax on muscle, and so the Eskimos live largely on the *blubber and fat of aquatic animals.* No other diet is possible to them; they could not get fruits, nuts, or vegetables even if they were disposed to eat them; and they could not live on them in that climate if they could get them. So, notwithstanding the arguments of the vegetarians, the Eskimos will continue to live on animal fats.

On the other hand, as we come toward the TROPICS, we find fuel foods less required; and we find the people naturally inclining toward a *vegetarian diet.* Millions live on rice and fruits; and the food regimen of an Eskimo village, if followed upon the equator, would result in speedy death. A "natural" diet for the equatorial regions would be very far from being a natural diet near the North Pole. The people of either zone, if not interfered with by medical or dietary "scientists," will be guided by the All-Intelligence, which seeks the fullest life in all, to feed themselves in the best way for the promotion of perfect health. In general, you can see that God, working in nature and in the evolution of human society and customs, has answered your question as to what you will eat. We advise you to take His answer in preference to that of any person.

In the TEMPERATE ZONE, the largest demands are made upon people's spirit, mind, and body; and here we find the greatest variety of foods provided by Nature. It is really quite useless and superfluous to theorize on the question as to what the masses will eat, for they have no choice — they must eat the foods which are staple products of the zone in which they live. It is impossible to supply all the people with a nut-and-fruit or raw-food diet. The fact that it is impossible is proof positive these are not the foods intended for the temperate zone by Nature. For Nature, being formed for the advancement of life, has never prohibited us from food, or the very means which sustain life.

So, as to the question in the TEMPERATE ZONE, "What will I eat?" The answer is quite clear: *Eat wheat, corn, rye, oats, barley, buckwheat; eat vegetables; eat meats; eat fruits; eat the things that are eaten by the masses of the people around the* world. In this matter, the voice of people is the voice of the Supreme. They have been led, generally, to the selection of certain foods; and

If you do not eat until you have an EARNED hunger, you will not find your tastebuds demanding unnatural or unhealthy foods.

they have been led, generally, to prepare these foods in generally similar ways; and you may assume that, in general, they have the right foods and are preparing them in the right way. In these matters the race in the temperate zone has been under the guidance of God. The list of foods in common use is a long one, and you must select from this list according to your individual taste; if you do, you will find you have an infallible guide, as shown in the next two chapters.

If you do not eat until you have an EARNED hunger, you will not find your tastebuds demanding unnatural or unhealthy foods. The carpenter, who has swung his or her hammer continuously from seven in the morning until noon does not come in clamoring for cream puffs and confectionery. This individual wants pork and beans, or beefsteak and potatoes, or corned beef and cabbage; they ask for the plain solids. Offer to crack them a few walnuts and give them a plate of lettuce, and you will be met with great argument; those things are not natural foods for a working person. And if they are not natural foods for a working person, they are not for any other individual — for *work-hunger is the only real hunger*. It requires the same materials to satisfy it, whether it be in bus driver or banker, in man, woman, or child.

It is a mistake to suppose food must be selected with anxious care to fit the vocation of the person who consumes it. The truth is, the carpenter does not require "heavy" or "solid" foods, and the bookkeeper "light" foods. If you are a bookkeeper, or other brain-worker, and do not eat until you have an EARNED hunger, you will want exactly the same foods the carpenter wants. Your body is made of exactly the same elements as that of the carpenter, and requires the same materials for cell-building. Why, then, feed the carpenter on ham and eggs and corn bread, and you on crackers and toast? True, most of their waste is of muscle, while most of yours is of brain and nerve tissue; but it is also true the carpenter's diet contains all the requisites for brain and nerve building in far better proportions than they are found in most "light" foods. The world's best brain-work has been done on the food of the working people.

> *Indigestion is never caused by eating to satisfy hunger; it is always caused by eating to gratify appetite.*

The world's greatest thinkers have invariably lived on the plain solid foods common among the masses.

Let the bookkeeper wait until they have an earned hunger before they eat; and then, if they want ham, eggs, and corn bread, by all means, let them eat it. But let them remember, they do not need one-twentieth of the amount necessary for the carpenter. It is not eating "hearty" foods which gives the brain-worker indigestion; it is eating as much as would be needed by a muscle-worker.

Indigestion is never caused by eating to satisfy hunger; it is always caused by eating to gratify appetite. If you eat in the manner prescribed in the next chapter, your taste will soon become so natural, you will never WANT anything you cannot eat with impunity; and you can drop the whole anxious question of what to eat from your mind forever, and simply eat what you want. Indeed, this

If you want pie, cake, pastry or puddings, it is better to begin your meal with them, finishing with the plainer and less tasty foods.

method is the only way to follow if you are thinking of no thoughts but those of health... for you cannot think health so long as you are in continual doubt and uncertainty as to whether you are eating the right foods, and getting the right nutrients.

The habit of eating purely for sensual gratification is very deeply-rooted within most of us. The usual "dessert" of sweet and tempting foods is prepared solely with a view to induce people to eat after hunger has been satisfied; and all the effects are ill-producing. It is not that pie and cake are unwholesome foods; they are usually perfectly wholesome if eaten to satisfy hunger, and NOT to gratify appetite. *If you want pie, cake, pastry or puddings, it is better to begin your meal with them, finishing with the plainer and less tasty foods.* You will find, however, that if you eat as we have directed, the plainest food will soon come to taste like kingly fare to you; for your sense of taste, like all your other senses, will become so acute with the general improvement in your condition, you will find new delights in common things. No glutton ever enjoyed a meal like the person who eats for hunger only, who gets the most out of every mouthful, and who stops on the instant they feel the edge

If you wish to be exactly and rigidly scientific, drink nothing but water; drink only when you are thirsty; drink whenever you are thirsty, and stop as soon as you feel that your thirst begins to abate.

taken from their hunger. The first intimation that hunger is abating is the signal from the inner-conscious mind saying it is time to quit.

WHAT TO DRINK

The matter of drinking in a natural way may be addressed here with a very few words. If you wish to be exactly and rigidly scientific, *drink nothing but water; drink only when you are thirsty;* drink whenever you are thirsty, and stop as soon as you feel your thirst quenched. But if you are living rightly in regard to eating, it will not be necessary to practice abstinence or great self-denial in the matter of drinking. You can take an occasional cup of weak coffee without harm; you can, to a reasonable extent, follow the customs of those around you. Do not get the soda-pop habit; do not drink merely to tickle your palate with sweet liquids. Be sure you take a drink of water whenever you feel thirsty.

Never be too lazy, too indifferent, or too busy to get a drink of water when you feel the very least thirst; if you obey this rule, you will have little inclination to take strange and unnatural drinks. Drink only to satisfy thirst; drink whenever you feel thirst; and stop drinking as soon as you feel thirst abating. This replenishment is the perfectly healthy way to supply the food with the necessary fluid material for its internal processes.

SUMMARY

As to what you will eat, you must be guided by Intelligence which has arranged the people of any given portion of the earth's surface to live on the staple products of the zone which they inhabit. Have faith in Intelligence, and ignore "food science" of every kind. Do not pay the slightest attention to the controversies as to the relative merits of cooked and raw foods; of vegetables and meats; or as to your need for carbohydrates, proteins, and fats.

It is not necessary to worry about a "varied" diet, so as to get in all the necessary elements. The Chinese and Hindus build very good bodies and excellent brains on a diet of few variations, rice making up almost the whole of it. The Scots are physically and mentally strong on oatmeal cakes; and the Irish are husky of body and brilliant of mind on potatoes and pork. The wheat berry contains practically all that is necessary for the building of brain and body; and a person can live very well on a mono-diet of navy beans.

Form a Conception of Perfect Health for yourself, and do not hold any thought which is not a thought of health.

NEVER eat until you have an EARNED HUNGER. Remember, it will not hurt you in the least to go hungry for a short time; but it will surely hurt you to eat when you are not hungry. Eat the common foods of the masses of the people in the zone in which you live, and have perfect confidence that the results will be good. They will be. Do not seek for luxuries, or for things imported or fixed up to tempt the taste; stick to plain solids; and when these do not "taste good," fast until they do. Do not seek for "light" foods; eat what the farmers and workers eat. Then you will be functioning in a perfectly healthy manner, so far as what to eat is concerned.

If you have no hunger or taste for the plain foods, do not eat at all; wait until hunger comes. Go without eating until the plainest food tastes good to you; and then *begin your meal with what you like best.*

We repeat, do not give the least thought to what you should or should not eat; simply eat what is set before you, selecting what pleases your taste most. In other words, eat what you want. This you can do with perfect results if you eat in the Right Way; and how to do this will be explained in the next chapter.

CHAPTER TEN

HOW TO EAT

*T*his is a settled fact that humans naturally chew their food. And if it is natural we should chew our food, the more thoroughly we chew it, the more completely natural the process must be. If you will chew every mouthful to a liquid, you need not be in the least concerned as to what you will eat, for you can get sufficient nourishment out of any ordinary food.

> Whether or not this chewing will be an irksome and laborious task or a most enjoyable process, depends upon the mental attitude in which you come to the table.

If your mind and attitude are on other things, or if you are anxious or worried about business or family affairs, you will find it almost impossible to eat without bolting more or less of your food. You must learn to live so scientifically that you will have no business or domestic cares to worry about. This you can do (read *The Science of Getting Rich* and *The Science of Becoming Excellent*), and you can also learn to give your undivided attention to the act of eating, while at the table.

When you eat, focus on the purpose of getting all the enjoyment you can from that meal. Dismiss everything else from your mind, and do not let anything take your attention from the food and its taste until your meal is finished. Be cheerfully confident, for if you follow these instructions, you may KNOW the food you eat is exactly the right food, and it will "agree" with you to perfection.

✳ Do not eat standing up, while driving a car, or while watching television. Sit down to the table with confident cheerfulness, and take a moderate portion of the food; take whatever looks most desirable to you.

✳ Do not select some food because you think it will be good for you; select edibles which will taste good to you. If you are to get well and stay well, you must drop the idea of doing things because they are good for your health, and do things because you want to do them. Select the food you want most; gratefully give thanks to God that you have learned how to eat it in such a way for digestion to be perfect; and take a moderate mouthful of it.

✳ Do not fix your attention on the act of chewing; fix it on the TASTE of the food; and taste and enjoy it until it is reduced to a liquid state and passes down your throat by involuntary swallowing. No matter how long it takes — CHEW — do not think of the time... *think of the taste.*

❋ Do not allow your eyes to wander over the table, speculating as to what you will eat next; do not worry for fear there is not enough, and you will not get your share of everything.

❋ Do not anticipate the taste of the next thing; keep your mind centered on the taste of what you have in your mouth. And that is all you need to focus on.

Scientific and healthful eating is a delightful process after you have learned how to do it, and after you have overcome the harmful old habit of gobbling down your food unchewed. It is best not to have too much conversation going on while eating; be cheerful, but not talkative; do the talking afterward. (Talking forces you to swallow food unchewed... so you can get in on the conversation!)

In most cases, some use of the will is required to form the habit of correct eating. The bolting or "gobbling" habit is an unnatural one, and is without doubt mostly the result of:

✳ 1. FEAR: a) fear that we will be robbed of our food; b) fear that we will not get our share of the good things; c) fear that we will lose precious time — these are the causes of haste.

✳ 2. Then there is ANTICIPATION of the goodies that are to come *for dessert*, and the consequent desire to get at them as quickly as possible. And there is;

✳ 3. MENTAL ABSTRACTION, or thinking of other matters while eating. All these must be overcome.

When you find your mind wandering, call a halt; think for a moment of the food, and of how good it tastes; of the perfect digestion and assimilation which is going to follow the meal, and begin again. Begin again and again, though you must do so twenty times in the course of a single meal; and again and again, though you must do so every meal for weeks and months. It is perfectly certain you CAN form the scientific eating habit if you persevere; and when you have formed it, you will experience a healthful pleasure you have never known.

Say mentally to yourself, while placing your hands over the food you are about to eat...

"All the food I am to eat, my body will naturally digest and assimilate the vitamins and nutrients it needs... and the remainder will be eliminated easily from my body. I am grateful."

This is a vital point, and we must not leave it until we have thoroughly impressed it upon your mind. *Given the right materials, perfectly prepared, the Principle of Health will positively build you a perfectly healthy body*; and you cannot prepare the materials perfectly in any other way than the one we are describing. If you are to have perfect health, you MUST eat in just this way; you can, and doing it is only a matter of a little perseverance.

What is the use for you to talk of mental control unless you will govern yourself in so simple a matter as ceasing to bolt your food? What's the use to talk of concentration unless you can keep your mind on the act of eating for so short a space as fifteen or twenty minutes, especially with all the pleasures of taste to help you? Go on, and conquer. In a couple of weeks, or months, as the case may be, you will find the habit of *scientific eating* becoming fixed; and soon you will be in so ex-

> *Given the right materials, perfectly prepared, the Principle of Health will positively build you a perfectly healthy body...*

cellent a condition, mentally and physically, that nothing would induce you to return to the harming old way.

HOW MUCH TO EAT

It is very easy to find the correct answer to the question, How much will I eat? *You are never to eat until you have an earned hunger, and you are to stop eating the instant you BEGIN to feel your hunger is abating.* Never gorge yourself; never eat to excess. When you begin to feel that your hunger is satisfied, know that you have enough; for until you have enough, you will continue to feel the sensation of hunger. If you eat as previously directed, it is probable you will begin to feel satisfied before you have taken half your usual amount; but stop there, all the same. No matter how delightfully attractive the dessert, or how tempting the pie or

> The amount of food required depends upon the work; upon how much muscular exercise is taken, and upon the extent to which the person is exposed to cold.

pudding, do not eat a mouthful of it if you find your hunger has been in the least degree assuaged by the other foods you have taken.

Whatever you eat after your hunger begins to abate is taken to gratify taste and appetite, not hunger and is not called for by nature at all. It is therefore excess; mere corruption, and it cannot fail but work mischief.

The average person who takes up this scientific plan of living will be greatly surprised to learn how little food is really required to keep the body in perfect condition. The amount of food required depends upon the work; upon how much muscular exercise is taken, and upon the extent to which the person is exposed to cold. The logger who goes into the forest in the winter time and swings his axe all day can eat two full meals; but the brain-worker who sits all day on a chair, in a warm room, does not need one-third and often not one-tenth as much. Most loggers eat two or three times as much, and most brain-workers from three to ten times as much as nature calls for; and *the elimination of this vast amount of surplus rubbish from their systems is a tax on vital power which, in time, depletes their energy and leaves them an easy prey to so-called disease.* Get all possible enjoyment out of the taste of your food, but never eat anything merely because it tastes good; and on the instant you feel that your hunger is less keen, stop eating.

If you will consider for a moment, you will see there is positively no other way for you to settle these various food questions than by adopting the plan here laid down for you.

DEVELOP A HEALTHY ATTITUDE

The importance of the mental attitude is sufficient to justify an additional word. While you are eating, as well as other times, think only of healthy conditions and normal functioning. Enjoy what you eat; if you carry on a conversation at the table, talk of the goodness of the food, and of the pleasure it is giving you. Never mention you dislike this or that; speak only of those things which you like. Never discuss the wholesomeness or unwhole-

> *Let your watchword be perseverance; whenever you fall into the old way of hasty eating, or of wrong thought and speech, bring yourself up short and begin again.*

someness of foods; never mention or think of unwholesomeness at all. If there is anything on the table for which you do not care, pass it by in silence, without a word or comment; never criticize or object to anything. Eat your food with gladness and singleness of heart, praising God and giving thanks. Let your watchword be perseverance; whenever you fall into the old way of hasty eating, or of wrong thought and speech, bring yourself up short and begin again. The crucial part of well-being is maintaining the system of healthy thoughts and actions. If you fall backward, be sure your next step is forward — improve! Don't let a mistake become an all-encompassing habit!

It is of the most vital importance to you to become a *self-controlling* and *self-directing* person; and you can never hope to become so unless you can master yourself in so simple and fundamental a matter as the manner and method of your eating. If you cannot control yourself in this aspect, you cannot control yourself in anything that will be worthwhile. On the other hand, if you carry out the foregoing instructions, you may rest in the assurance that in so far as right thinking and right eating are concerned, you are living in a perfectly Scientific Way. You may also be assured that if you practice what is prescribed in the following chapters you will quickly build your body into a condition of perfect health.

The success in anything is attained by making each separate act a success in itself. If you make each action (however small and unimportant), a thoroughly successful action, your day's work as a whole cannot result in failure. If you make the actions of each day successful, the sum total of your life cannot be failure. A great success is the result of doing a large number of little things, and doing each one in a perfectly successful way. If every thought is a healthy thought, and if every action of your life is performed in a healthy way, you must soon attain to perfect health.

It is impossible to devise a more logical way to perform the act of eating more successfully, and in a manner more in accord with the laws of life, than by chewing every mouthful to a liquid, enjoying the taste fully, and keeping a cheerful confidence all the while. Nothing can be added to make the process more successful; while if anything be subtracted, the process will not be a completely healthy one.

Q. What will I do about the great bugaboo which scares millions of people to death every year — Constipation?

A. Do nothing. When you live on this scientific plan you need not, and indeed cannot, have an evacuation of the bowels every day; and that an operation in from once in two days to twice a week is quite sufficient for perfect health. The gross feeders who eat from three to ten times as much as can be utilized in their systems have a great amount of waste to eliminate (and therefore, Nature has the challenge of evacuating it from their body... before they stuff in more!). But if you live in the manner we have described, it will be different with you.

If you eat only when you have an EARNED HUNGER, and chew every mouthful to a liquid, and if you stop eating the instant you BEGIN to be conscious of an abatement of your hunger, you will so perfectly prepare your food for digestion and assimilation that practically all of it will be taken up by the bloodstream; and there will be little — almost nothing — remaining in the bowels to be excreted. If you are able to entirely banish from your memory all that you have read in "doctor books" and patent medicine advertisements concerning constipation, you need give the matter no further thought at all. The *Principle of Health* will take care of it.

But if your mind has been filled with fear-thoughts in regard to constipation, it may be well in the beginning for you to occasionally flush the colon with warm water. There is not the least need of doing it, except to make the process of your mental emancipation from fear a little easier; it may be worthwhile for that. And as soon as you see you are making good progress, and you have cut down your quantity of food, and are really eating in the Scientific Way, dismiss constipation from your mind forever; you have nothing more to do with it. Put your trust in that Principle within you which has the power to give you perfect health; relate to It by your reverent gratitude to the Principle of Life which is All Power, and go on your way rejoicing.

SUMMARY

In the matter of how much to eat, you must be guided by the same inward Intelligence, or *Principle of Health*, which indicates when food is wanted. You must stop eating the moment that you feel hunger abating; you must not eat beyond this point to gratify taste. If you cease to eat in the instant when the inward demand for food ceases, you will *never* overeat; and the function of supplying the body with food will be performed in a perfectly healthy manner.

Hunger is never a disagreeable feeling, accompanied by weakness, faintness, or gnawing feelings at the stomach; it is a pleasant, anticipatory desire for food, and is felt mostly in the mouth and throat. It does not come at certain hours or at stated intervals; it only comes when the inner-conscious mind is ready to receive, digest, and assimilate food.

The matter of eating naturally is a very simple one; there is nothing in all the foregoing which cannot be easily practiced by anyone. This method, put in practice, will infallibly result in perfect chemistry for digestion and assimilation; and all anxiety and careful thought concerning the matter can at once be dropped from the mind. Once your mental thoughts are not so focused on what to eat, how much to eat, and when to eat — the rest of your faculties will be able to develop and flourish.

Eat your food with cheerful confidence, and get all the pleasure to be had from the taste of every mouthful. Chew each morsel to a liquid, keeping your attention fixed on the enjoyment of the process. This practice is the only way to eat in a perfectly complete and successful manner; and when anything is done in a completely successful manner, the general result cannot be a failure. In the attainment of health, the Law is the same as in the attainment of riches; if you make each act a success in itself, the sum of all your acts must be a success. When you eat in the mental attitude we have prescribed, and in the manner we have described, nothing can be added to the process; it is done in a perfect manner, and it is successfully begun.

PART III

BREATHE AND SLEEP YOURSELF TO PERFECT HEALTH

CHAPTER ELEVEN

THE BREATH OF LIFE

*T*he function of breathing is a vital one, and directly concerns the continuance of life. We can live many hours without sleeping, and many days without eating or drinking, but only a few minutes without breathing. The act of breathing is involuntary, but the manner of it, and the provision of the proper conditions for its healthy performance, falls within the scope of volition. You will continue to breathe involuntarily, but

> *You will continue to breathe involuntarily, but you can voluntarily determine what you will breathe, and how deeply and thoroughly you will breathe.*

you can voluntarily determine what you will breathe, and how deeply and thoroughly you will breathe. You can, of your own volition, keep the physical mechanism in condition for the perfect performance of the function.

Although well-equipped with two lungs, most people seldom fill either of them with life propelling oxygen, and even still, abuse them with smoke. It is essential, if you wish to breathe in a perfectly healthy way, that the physical machinery used in the act should be kept in good condition. You must keep your spine moderately straight, and the muscles of your chest must be flexible and free in action. You cannot breathe in the right way if your shoulders are greatly stooped forward and your chest hollow and rigid. Sitting or standing at work in a slightly stooping position tends to produce hollow chest; so does lifting heavy or light weights.

The tendency in work, of almost all kinds, is to pull the shoulders forward, curve the spine, and flatten the chest — and if the chest is greatly flattened, full and deep breathing becomes impossible, and perfect health is out of the question.

Various gymnastic exercises have been devised to counteract the effect of stooping while at work; such as hanging by the hands from a swing or trapeze bar, or sitting on a chair with the feet under some heavy article of furniture and bending backward until the head touches the floor, and so on. And all the aerobic exercises are good enough in their own way, but very few people will follow them long enough and regularly enough to accomplish any real gain in physique. The taking on of "health exercise" of any kind is burdensome and unnecessary; there is a more natural, simpler, and more effective way.

This better way is to keep yourself straight, and to breathe deeply. Let your mental conception of yourself be that you are a perfectly straight person, and whenever the matter comes to your mind, be sure you instantly expand your chest, throw back your shoulders, and "straighten up." Whenever you do this, slowly draw in your breath until you fill your lungs to their utmost capacity; "crowd in" all the air you possibly can. While holding it for an instant in the lungs, throw your shoulders still further back, and stretch your chest; at the same time try to pull your spine forward between the shoulders. Then exhale the air easily.

This technique is the one great exercise for keeping the chest full, flexible, and in good condition: Straighten up; fill your lungs FULL; stretch your chest and straighten your spine, and exhale easily.

✳ Don't slouch, don't slump, don't sag, don't droop.

✳ Sit straight, stand straight, talk straight, act straight.

You must repeat this exercise, in season and out of season, at all times and in all places, until you form a habit of doing it; you can easily do so. Whenever you step out of doors into the fresh air, BREATHE. When you are at work, and think of yourself and your position, BREATHE. When you are in company, and are reminded of the matter, BREATHE. When you are awake, even in the middle of the night, BREATHE. No matter where you are or what you are doing, whenever the idea comes to your mind, straighten up and BREATHE. If you walk to and from your work, take the exercise all the way; it will soon become a delight to you; you will keep it up, not for the sake of health, but as a matter of pleasure.

A correct posture is essential to a strong, and confident personality. To help in this manner, you can occasionally do the following exercise: Once in a while, stand up, clasp your hands behind your back, bringing them well up between the shoulder blades, then take a full, deep breath, expanding the chest to its capacity, at the same time straightening the arms while keeping the hands clasped. This is a great exercise for developing erect posture.

Simple, natural breathing promotes good health, and extends life. And the best way to promote the deep breathing in of Life is to walk outdoors. A brisk walk, in all kinds of weather, pays high dividends. It leads to greater efficiency of movement and less fatigue, caused by lack of oxygen; lack of connection to the Source.

Learn how to walk properly, with a free, easy stepping stride, carrying the weight of the body on the muscles, and not on the bones. To stay youthful, walk erect by lifting the body to its fullest length. This is one way to use (and, therefore, bring Life Force to and oxygenate) all the muscles from your neck down to your feet.

Do not consider these "health exercises," never do health exercises, or do gymnastics, or aerobics to make yourself well. To do so is to recognize sickness as a present fact or as a possibility, which is precisely what you must not do!

✳ Walking promotes sleep, rest, and relaxation of mind, body, and spirit.

✳ Walking exercises the mind, and drives away the cobwebs.

✳ Walking exercises the emotions, and gives you an opportunity to observe and enjoy the world.

✳ Walking uplifts the spirit, as you exhale human body tensions and breathe in the power of the Source.

Do not consider these "health exercises," never do health exercises, or do gymnastics, or aerobics to make yourself well. To do so is to recognize sickness as a present fact or as a possibility, which is precisely what you must not do! The people who are always doing exercises for their health are always thinking about being sick. *It ought to be a matter of pride with yourself to keep your spine straight and strong;* as much so as it is to keep your face clean. Keep your spine straight, and your chest full and flexible for the same reason that you keep your hands clean and your nails manicured... because it is lazy to do otherwise. Do it without a thought of sickness, present or possible. You must either be crooked and unsightly, or you must be straight; and if you are straight your breathing will take care of itself.

It is essential, however, that you should breathe AIR. It appears to be the intention of Nature that the lungs should receive air containing its regular percentage of oxygen, and not greatly contaminated by other gases, or by filth of any kind. Do not allow yourself to think you are compelled to live or work where the air is not fit to breathe. If your house cannot be properly ventilated, move. If you are employed where the air is bad, get another job (you can, by practicing the methods given in the preceding volume of this series *The Science of Getting Rich).* If no one would consent to work in bad air, employers would speedily see to it that all work rooms were properly ventilated.

This technique is the one great exercise for keeping the chest full, flexible, and in good condition: Straighten up; fill your lungs FULL; stretch your chest and straighten your spine, and exhale easily.

The worst air is that from which the oxygen has been exhausted by breathing; as that of churches and theaters where crowds of people congregate, and the outlet and supply of air are poor. Next to this poor air is air containing gases other than oxygen — hydrogen-sewer gas, and the fumes from decaying things. Air that is heavily charged with dust or particles of organic matter may be endured better than any of these. Small particles of organic matter other than food are generally thrown-off from the lungs... but gases go into the blood. See to it you do not breathe air containing poisonous gases, and you do not inhale the air which has been used by yourself or others.

Air is largely a food. It is the most thoroughly alive thing we take into the body. *Every breath carries within it millions of microbes, many of which are assimilated.* The odors from earth, grass, tree, flower, plant, and from cooking foods are nourishments in themselves. These odors contain minute particles of the substances from which they come, and are often so small they pass directly from the lungs into the bloodstream, and are assimilated without digestion.

> *Air is largely a food. It is the most thoroughly alive thing we take into the body. Every breath carries within it millions of microbes, many of which are assimilated.*

The atmosphere is permeated with the one Original Substance, which is life itself! Consciously recognize this whenever you think of your breathing, and think that you are breathing in life — you really are, and conscious recognition helps the process. (The breathing in of Original Substance during exercise is the one true reason as to their possible positive effects.) Therefore, fill your lungs full and deep of life! Disregard sickness and unhealthy elements — internally and externally.

Q. What about exercise?

A. Everyone is the better for a little all-around use of the muscles every day; and the best way to get this activity is to do it by engaging in some form of play or amusement. Get your exercise in

> *The atmosphere is permeated with the one Original Substance, which is life itself!*

the natural way; as recreation, not as a forced stunt for health's sake alone. Ride a horse or a bicycle; play tennis or bowling, or toss a ball. Have some hobby like gardening in which you can spend an hour every day with pleasure and profit. There are a thousand ways in which you can get exercise enough to keep your body supple and your circulation good, and yet not fall into the rut of "exercising for your health." *Exercise for fun or profit; exercise because you are too healthy to sit still, and not because you wish to become healthy, or to remain so.*

SUMMARY

With every fresh breath of air inhaled, a miracle takes place. The poison-filled blue blood which enters the lungs is charged with the life-giving air which you breath. It is instantly purified and given new life. New blood — rich, pure, red — flows to all parts of your body, bringing with it NEW LIFE. Breathe in sufficient oxygen to burn-up dead, broken-down tissue, and to keep your bloodstream clean and strong.

That is all there is to the matter of breathing correctly — keep your spine straight and your chest flexible, and breathe pure air. Hold yourself erect and dignified. Recognize with thankfulness, the fact that you breathe in the Eternal Life. This idea is not difficult; and beyond these things give little thought to your breathing except to thank the Source that you have learned how to do it perfectly. Be thankful for the Breath of Life and Its wonderful effect to revitalize, renew, and restore your body.

CHAPTER TWELVE

SLEEP TO RENEW THE SPIRIT

*V*ital power is renewed in sleep. Every living thing sleeps; men, animals, reptiles, fish, and insects sleep, and even plants have regular periods of slumber. And this is because it is in sleep that you come into such contact with the Principle of Life in nature, which allows your own life to be renewed. It is the time when you submit yourself lovingly and completely to Nature. It is in sleep your brain is recharged with vital energy, and the

> *... in sleep that we come into such contact with the Principle of Life in nature that our own lives may be renewed. It is in sleep that your brain is recharged with vital energy, and the Principle of Health within you is given new strength.*

Principle of Health within you is given new strength. It is of the first importance, then, you should sleep in a natural, normal, and perfectly healthy manner.

Approximately one-third of our natural lives are spent in sleep, yet it is surprising to learn most people have not learned the art of *restful* sleeping.

Studying sleep, we note that the breathing is much deeper, and more forcible and rhythmic than in the waking state. Much more air is inhaled when asleep than when awake. This fact tells us that the *Principle of Health* requires large quantities of some element in the atmosphere for the process of renewal. If you would surround sleep with natural conditions, then:

> ✳ *STEP 1: the first step is to see that you have an unlimited supply of fresh and pure air to breathe.*

Physicians have found that sleeping in the pure outdoor air is very efficacious in the treatment of pulmonary troubles. Taken in connection with the Way of Living and Thinking prescribed in this book, you will find it is just as effective in curing every other sort of trouble.

Do not take any halfway measures in this matter of securing pure air while you sleep. *Ventilate your bedroom thoroughly*; so thoroughly it will be practically the same as sleeping outdoors. Have a door or window open wide; have one open on each side of the room, if possible. If you cannot have a good draft of air across the room, pull the head of your bed close to the open window, so the air from outside may come fully into your face. No matter how cold or unpleasant the weather, have an open window, and open it widely; try to get a circulation of pure air throughout the room. Pile on the blankets, if necessary, to keep you warm; but have an unlimited supply of fresh air from outdoors. This is the first great requisite for healthy sleep.

The brain and nerve centers cannot be thoroughly vitalized if you sleep in "dead" or stagnant air — you must have the living atmosphere, vital with nature's *Principle of Life*. We repeat, do not make any compromise in this matter; ventilate your sleeping room completely, and see that there is a circulation of outdoor air through it while you sleep. You are not sleeping in a perfectly healthy way if you shut the doors and windows of your sleeping room, whether in winter or summer. Have fresh air. If you are where there is no fresh air, move. If your bedroom cannot be ventilated, get into another house.

> ✳ *STEP 2: Next in importance is the mental attitude in which you go to sleep. It is well to sleep intelligently, purposefully, knowing what you do it for.*

Lie down thinking that sleep is an infallible vitalizer, and go to sleep with a confident faith your strength is to be renewed; think you will awaken full of vitality and health. *Put purpose into your sleep as you do into your eating; give the matter your attention for a few minutes, as you go to rest.* Do no seek your bed with a discouraged or depressed feeling; go there joyously, to be made whole. Read inspirational material before going to sleep — never go to bed with a negative news broadcast on your mind. Keep your mind fresh, pure and with cheerful thoughts before dropping off to sleep. *Never go to bed mentally tired.*

Do not forget the exercise of gratitude in going to sleep. Before you close your eyes, give thanks to God for having shown you the way to perfect health, and go to sleep with this grateful thought uppermost in your mind. A bedtime prayer or meditation of thanksgiving is a well-thought effort; it puts the *Principle of Health* within you into communication with its Source, from which It is to receive new power while you are in the silence of unconsciousness.

> *A bedtime prayer or meditation of thanksgiving is a well-thought effort; it puts the Principle of Health within you into comm-unication with its Source, from which It is to receive new power while you are in the silence of unconsciousness.*

SUMMARY

Periods of relaxation, rest, and sleep are absolutely essential for the maintenance of good physical health. When you go to bed, just like hanging up your clothes... hang up any business or personal troubles and tensions.

You may see the requirements for perfectly healthy sleep are not difficult: 1) to see you breathe pure air from outdoors while you sleep; and, 2) to put the Within in touch with the Living Substance by a few minutes of grateful meditation as you go to bed.

Observe these requirements, go to sleep in a thankful and confident frame of mind, and all will be well. If you have INSOMNIA, do not let it worry you. While you lie awake, form your Conception of Health; meditate with thankfulness on the abundant life which is yours, breathe, and feel perfectly confident you will sleep in due time; and you will. Insomnia, like every other ailment, must give way before the *Principle of Health*, aroused to full constructive activity by the course of thought and action described here.

You can now comprehend it is not at all burdensome or disagreeable to perform the voluntary functions of life in a perfectly healthy way. The perfectly healthy way is the easiest, simplest, most natural, and most pleasant way. The cultivation of health is not a work of art, difficult, or strenuous labor. You have only to lay aside artificial observances of every kind, and eat, drink, breathe, and sleep in the most natural and delightful way. If you live in this manner, thinking health and only health, you will certainly be well.

SUMMARY

TRUTHS TO
THE SCIENCE OF WELL-BEING

Health is perfectly natural functioning, normal living. There is a *Principle of Life* in the Universe; it is the Living Substance, from which all things are made. This Living Substance permeates, penetrates, and fills the interspaces of the universe. In its invisible state, it is in and through all forms; and yet all forms are made of it.

To illustrate: Suppose a very fine and highly diffusible aqueous vapor should permeate and penetrate a block of ice. The ice is formed from living water, and is living water in form; while the vapor is also living water, unformed, permeating a form made from itself. This illustration will explain how Living Substance permeates all forms made from It; all life comes from It; It is all the life there is.

This Universal Substance is a thinking substance, and takes the form of Its thought. The thought of a form, held by It, creates the form; and the thought of a motion causes the motion. It cannot help thinking, and so is forever creating; and It must move on toward fuller and more complete expression of Itself. This movement is toward a more complete life and more perfect functioning; and that means toward perfect health.

The power of the Living Substance must always be exerted toward perfect health; It is a force in all things, making for perfect functioning.

All things are permeated by a power which makes for health. You can relate yourself to this Power and ally yourself with It; you can also separate yourself from It in your thoughts.

You are a form of this Living Substance, and have within you a *Principle of Health*. This *Principle of Health*, when in full constructive activity, causes all the *involuntary* functions of your body to be perfectly performed.

You are a thinking substance, permeating a visible body, and the processes of your body are controlled by your thought.

When you think only thoughts of perfect health, the internal processes of your body will be those of perfect health. Your first step toward perfect health must be to form a conception of yourself as a perfectly healthy person. Having formed this conception, you must relate yourself to it in all your thoughts, and sever all thought relations with disease and weakness

If you do this, and think your thoughts of health with positive FAITH, you will cause the *Principle of Health* within you to become constructively active, and to heal all your diseases. You can receive additional power from the Universal Principle of Life by faith, and you can acquire faith by looking to this Principle of Life with reverent gratitude for the health It gives you. If you will consciously accept the health which is being continually given to you by the Living Substance, and if you will be duly grateful therefore, you will develop faith.

Health is the result of thinking and acting in a Certain Way; and if a sick person begins to think and act in this Way, the *Principle of Health* within them will come into constructive activity and heal all the diseases. This *Principle of Health* is the same in all, and is related to the Life Principle of the Universe. It is able to heal every disease, and will come into activity whenever a person thinks and acts in accordance with *The Science of Well-Being.* Therefore, everyone can attain to perfect health!

You cannot think only thoughts of perfect health unless you perform the *voluntary functions* of life in a perfectly healthy manner. These voluntary functions are eating, drinking, breathing, and sleeping. If you think only thoughts of health, have faith in health, and eat, drink, breathe, and sleep in a perfectly healthy way, you must have perfect health.

In order to think only of healthy conditions and functioning, you must perform the voluntary acts of life in a perfectly healthy way. You cannot think perfect health so long as you know you are living in an unfit or unhealthy way; or even so long as you have doubts as to whether or not you are living in a healthy way. You cannot think thoughts of perfect health while your voluntary functions are performed in the manner of one who is sick. The voluntary functions of life are eating, drinking, breathing, and sleeping. When your thoughts are only of healthy conditions and functioning, and you are externally performing them in a perfectly healthy manner, you must have perfect health.

In eating, you must learn to be guided by your hunger. You must distinguish between hunger and appetite, and between hunger and the cravings of habit; you must NEVER eat unless you feel an EARNED HUNGER. You must learn genuine hunger is never present after natural sleep, and the demand for an early morning meal is purely a matter of habit and appetite; and you must not begin your day by eating in violation of Natural Law. You must wait until you have an earned hunger, which, in most cases, will make your first meal come at about the noon hour. No matter what your condition, vocation, or circumstance, you must make it your rule not to eat until you have an EARNED HUNGER; and you may remember it is far better to fast for several hours than to eat when your body is not in need nor prepared to handle food.

In deciding how to eat, you must be guided by reason. We can see that the abnormal states of hurry and worry produced by wrong thinking about business and similar things have led you to form the *habit of eating too fast, and chewing too little.* Reason tells us food should be chewed, and the more thoroughly it is chewed, the better it is prepared for the *chemistry of digestion.* Furthermore, we can see the person who eats slowly and chews their food to a liquid, keeping their mind on the process and giving it their undivided attention, will enjoy more of the pleasure of taste than one who bolts their food with their mind on something else.

To eat in a perfectly healthy manner, you must concentrate your attention on the act, with cheerful enjoyment and confidence; you must taste your food, and you must reduce each mouthful to a liquid before swallowing it. The foregoing instructions, if followed, make the function of eating completely perfect; nothing can be added as to what, when, and how.

Follow the instruction in *The Science of Well-Being...* activate the *Principle of Health...* and you will be healthy to enjoy an increase of Life!

The state of well-being in the most simplified thought: make yourself one with Health in thought, word, and action; and do not connect yourself with sickness either by thought, word, or action.

WALLACE D. WATTLES

*W*allace Wattles spent his entire life working out the principles and methods of the science outlined in this book. Through trial and error and much study and thought, he honed and polished his methods. In the final years of his life, using these principles and actions, he began to live in a state of well-being. He truly was a genius.

Born in the late 1800's, the major portion of his life was cursed by failures. Writes his daughter Florence, "He lost a good position in the Methodist Church because of his *heresy*. He met George D. Herron at a convention of reformers in Chicago in 1896 and caught Herron's social vision. From that day, until his death, he worked unceasingly to realize the glorious vision of human brotherhood."

Florence continues, "He wrote almost constantly... in his later years (while living in Elwood, Illinois). It was then that he formed his mental picture. He saw himself as a successful writer, a personality of power and health, an advancing man, and he began to work toward the realization of this vision... He lived every page of his books *(The Science of Getting Rich, The Science of Becoming Excellent, and The Science of Well-Being)*. His life was truly THE POWERFUL LIFE."

Wattles was a pioneer, and like the early trappers, he blazed the trails which became the freeways, in this case, to excellence and health.

DR. JUDITH POWELL

*D*r. Judith Powell knows that your real treasure lies hidden within, and she has shared her secrets with thousands in the U.S.A., Europe and the Orient.

An internationally sought-after authority and speaker on expanding human excellence, Judith has written definitive articles for business and the general community on numerous enlightening topics. She has also co-authored the self-improvement book, *Silva Mind Mastery For The '90s,* distributed worldwide and translated into seventeen languages. She is currently writing *A Date With Destiny,* a book on universal truths.

Judith's popular motivational seminars include: Color Dynamics, Loving Yourself, Discover Your Perfect Mate, Inner Power through Past Lives, Dreams and Destiny, An Introduction to Neuro Linguistic Programming, and Silva Mind Mastery. She also helps others find direction to excellence through her Mind Counseling.

After receiving her Bachelor's Degree in Color Design and Business at Marygrove College in Michigan, she earned her Master's and Doctorate Degrees in Psychorientology at the Institute of Psychorientology, Texas, as well as her Masters and Trainers Certifications in Neuro Linguistic Programming (the language of the brain).

Judith, an award-winning TV host for *It's All In Your Mind,* co-directs three companies in St. Petersburg, Florida with her husband, Dr. Tag Powell. They reside in the Tampa Bay area with their three Scottish Terriers — Master, Buddha, and Isis.

THE SCIENCE OF BECOMING EXCELLENT

Wallace D. Wattles and
Dr. Judith Powell

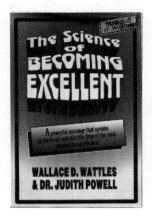

A timeless work that speaks to the heart and stirs the fires of the soul. It is second in the trilogy of answers. Where *The Science of Getting Rich* guides you to the KEYS of financial success, this writing supplies you with the solutions to a better future for reaching your peak potential. You hold your own Principle of Power. With awareness of this Principle, your mental faculties will be intelligently developed and purposely directed towards infinite greatness.

No person has yet become so great in any faculty where it is not possible for someone else to become greater! The plan of action laid down in this book will enable you to acknowledge and guide your growth potential toward true fulfillment. Life is too short to wait around for the world to effect you. YOU MUST AFFECT LIFE.

BONUS CHAPTER: EMERSON'S "OVERSOUL"

"You are designed to experience total completion. You are designed to be spiritually aware, mentally creative, emotionally well, physically vital, happy in relationships, and to be a goal-achiever."
—from Foreword by Roy Eugene Davis

ISBN 0-914295-96-9, 160 pages, $8.95 + $3.00s/h

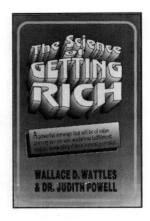

THE SCIENCE OF GETTING RICH

Wallace D. Wattles and Dr. Judith Powell

Fantastic: a down-to-earth, clear-cut and practical approach on "how to be rich." No bones about it, when you follow the thoughts presented in this book, you will become rich, without the feeling of guilt. The authors write that the poverty-stricken (and even the middle class) should feel guilty by not living up to their true potential as Thinking Beings. Attaining wealth has been written about many times over... along with a variety of programs for success, but when you read *this* rendition, you truly believe that *you* can do it! And after all, belief is the key to unlocking the door to success.

ISBN 1-56087-017-6, 160 pages, US $8.95 + $3.00s/h

RELAXING MUSIC — SUBLITONES®
by Peter Abood and Dr. Tag Powell

Sublitones®, researched for over ten years, is an ultra-effective behavior modification tool — *Mood Changers.*
Tuning the Rainbow — helps produce the feeling of *Security, Peace, Relaxation* and *Freedom from Stress.*

ISBN 0-914295-72-1 $9.95 + $3.00s/h

Charging the Body Electric — will give you *Courage* and *Strength* to help restore your *Self-Confidence.*

ISBN 0-914295-73-X $9.95 + $3.00s/h

Jazz Up Your Life — will help increase *Energy, Happiness, Enthusiasm* and *Stamina* to get the job done.

ISBN 0-914295-74-8 $9.95 + $3.00s/h

SILVA MIND MASTERY FOR THE '90s
by Dr. Tag Powell and Dr. Judith Powell

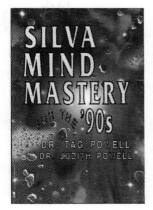

The how-to best-seller using the very latest research combined with the world's largest mind development training. Already translated into seventeen languages, the demand continues because of its practical applications and tools to easily improve your business and personal life. *Mind Mastery* covers: how to visualize, instant attitude adjustment, leadership skills, and creativity. Special techniques to improve relationships, sales, confidence, memory, and health. *Silva Mind Mastery for the '90s* will continue to empower you for years!
ISBN 0-914295-99-3, 256 pages, US $14.95 + $3.00s/h

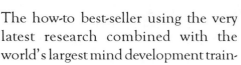

BALANCED LIVING SERIES
with Dr. Judith Powell

Enjoy the freedom of exploring and realizing your visions, dreams and ideals. Expand your true potential in all areas of your life. Includes: Financial Security, Social Confidence, Emotional Self-Control, Physical Well-Being, Personal Growth, Family Harmony, Spiritual Awareness, and Mental Power
In french-calf vinyl album, 8 Self-Improving Programs (8 audiocassettes), 8 Alphamatic Cards and Instruction Handbook.   *ISBN 0-914295-64-0 $79.95 + $8.00s/h*
(titles also sold separately at $9.95 +$3.00 s/h each)

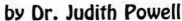